Dear Pharmacists,

S0-BWD-027

We are pleased to contribute to the publication of this reference tool, *The Practical Guide to Nonprescription Drugs*.

This new edition, researched and written by a dedicated team of pharmacists, is a rapid and efficient consultation tool to be used as a reference for patients inquiring about a health problem that can be treated with over-the-counter medication.

We hope that this guide will be useful in your daily practice. Please do not hesitate to communicate with your Pharmascience representative in order to obtain your copy or an additional copy.

Isabel Longval
Manager, Pharmacy Programs & Professional Relations - Quebec
Pharmascience Inc.

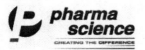

Table of Contents

Page

1. **Introduction**   1

2. **A Systematic Approach**   2

3. **Dermatological Problems**

Acne Vulgaris   4
Athlete's Foot   10
Burns   15
Chickenpox and Other Viral Skin Infections   22
Corns and Calluses of the Foot   29
Dandruff   33
Frostbite   37
Fungal Skin Infections   40
Insect Stings and Bites   46
Pruritus   52
Sun Protection   55
Sunburn   60
Warts   63

4. **Mouthcare**

Cold Sores   70
Dentin Hypersensitivity   74
Halitosis   76
Oral Ulcers   78
Thrush   83
Xerostomia   86

5. **Gastrointestinal Problems**

Constipation   90
Diarrhea   98
Dyspepsia   102
Gastroesophageal Reflux   110
Hemorrhoids   117
Intestinal Gas   122
Nausea and Vomiting   126
Preparing for a Diagnostic Test or for a Surgical Procedure   131

Table of Contents

Page

6. Parasites

Head Lice	138
Intestinal Worms	146
Pubic Lice	152
Scabies	154

7. Insomnia — 159

8. Ophthalmic Conditions

Blepharitis	166
Conjunctivitis	169
Contact Lens Care	176
Dry Eye	181
Styes	185

9. Ear Care

Cerumen Accumulation	189
Otitis Externa	193

10. Smoking Cessation — 196

11. Common Cold, Influenza, and Allergic Rhinitis — 208

12. Pain — 223

13. Women's Health

Dysmenorrhea	230
Emergency Contraception	234
Missed Hormonal Contraceptive	239
Osteoporosis	246
Vaginal Dryness	251
Vaginitis	255

Table of Contents

Page

14. Pediatric Care

Common Cold and Flu	263
Constipation	270
Fever and Febrile Seizures	279
Gastroenteritis	285
Infant Formulas and Nutrition	291
Infantile Colic	300
Teething Pain	303

15. Diagnostic Tests

Ovulation Tests	306
Pregnancy Tests	310

16. First-Aid Kits   314

17. Adjustment of Orthopedic Devices   318

18. Immunization Schedule   320

19. Pre-surgery Medication   332

20. Chronic Renal Failure and OTC Medication   336

21. Vitamins, Minerals, and Nutritional Supplements   340

22. Malnutrition and Nutritional Supplements   344

23. Sports Performance   352

24. Natural Products   362

25. Units of Measurement   389

26. Notes   390

Introduction

Introduction

Pharmacy shelves are filled with products and drugs that patients can use to prevent or quickly treat a great variety of health problems. The choice of an appropriate treatment, however, is difficult to make. *The Practical Guide to Nonprescription Drugs* was developed to help pharmacists respond quickly and effectively to numerous questions from patients.

This manual deals with frequently encountered problems and makes no claim to be exhaustive or comprehensive. Remember that your professional judgement remains your most dependable ally in dealing with more complex questions.

Good consulting!

The authors of the
The Practical Guide to Nonprescription Drugs

A Systematic Approach

A Systematic Approach

A systematic approach to the problem makes it possible to properly answer patients' questions and to make appropriate decisions about their health. These questions help the pharmacist obtain all the information needed to advise patients properly.

We therefore suggest the following approach:

1. Is it for you?

2. What are your symptoms?

3. How long have you had these symptoms?

4. What have you taken so far? Was it effective? Who advised this treatment?

5. Do you have any other health problems? What are they?

6. For women: Is there any possibility that you are pregnant? Are you breastfeeding?

7. Are you taking any medications (prescribed, OTC, natural products, vitamins) on a regular basis? Which ones?

8. Are you allergic to any medications? Which ones? What kind of allergic reaction?

Dermatological Problems

Acne Vulgaris

Acne Vulgaris

Questions to ask

✓ **How long have you had acne?**

✓ **Where are your lesions?**

✓ **How many lesions do you have?**

  ○ Only mild acne can be treated with over-the-counter products

Table I: Classification of Acne Vulgaris					
Severity	**Comedones**	**Papules/ Pustules**	**Nodules**	**Inflammation**	**Scars**
Mild	< 20	< 10	None	None	None
Moderate	> 20	10-20	+/-	+	None
Severe	> 20	> 20	> 10	++	+
Very severe	Large number	> 30	> 20	+++	+

- <u>Comedones</u>: commonly called blackheads or whiteheads
- <u>Papules</u>: (without pus) or pustules (with pus): small, solid, red elevations, usually < 5 mm in diameter
- <u>Nodules</u>: > 5 mm in diameter and deeper than papules or pustules

✓ **Which product do you use as a cleanser?**

✓ **Do you use any drugs regularly? (androgens, corticosteroids, lithium, oral contraceptives, topical products)?**

✓ **Is there anything that tends to aggravate your acne (makeup, hair products, wearing a cap or hairband, touching the lesions, menstrual cycle, seasonal changes, stress)?**

✓ **Is there a correlation between the appearance of the lesions and:**

- o beginning of menstruation?
- o adolescence?
- o pregnancy?

Table II: Medications That Could Cause or Exacerbate Acneiform Lesions	
Anabolic steroids	Azathioprine
Corticosteroids	Cyclosporine
Isoniazid	Disulfiram
Lithium	Phenobarbital
Phenytoin	Quinidine
Progestins	Vitamins B_1, B_6, B_{12}

What to do

Apply a light, fragrance-free moisturizing lotion for sensitive skin as needed to reduce skin irritation (e.g., *Cetaphil*)

- Choose water-based, greaseless, alcohol-free products
- Avoid touching the lesions
- Minimize stress factors
  - o There is no convincing evidence linking acne with diet
  - o Avoid physical irritants such as tight clothes, shirt collars, hair and hands touching your face
- Maintain good skin hygiene: wash twice a day, morning and evening, with a non-comedogenic product
  - o Use a neutral pH soap (*Dove*) or a non-irritating cleanser (see table below)
  - o Use soap substitutes (*Cetaphil*, *Tersaseptic*, *Spectro Jel*, La Roche-Posay {*Effaclar*}, *Johnson's pH 5.5*, *Avene* products)
  - o Avoid cream-based cleansers

Table III: Level of Irritation of Soaps or Detergent Bars		
Classification	**Soap**	**Level of Irritation**
Minimally irritating	*Dove*	0.5
Slightly irritating	*Aveeno*	2.2
	Dial	2.4
	Alpha Keri	2.5
	Neutrogena	2.8
	Ivory	2.8
	Oilatum	2.8
Irritating	*Jergens*	3.3
	Cuticara	3.9
	Irish Spring	4.0
	Zest	6.1
	Camay	6.4

Adapted from Québec Pharmacie 41(7), September 1994

What to use

- Re-evaluate the suggested treatment every six weeks

- Explain to the patient that the objective of the treatment is to prevent the appearance of new lesions and to avoid aggravating the existing lesions, because these will heal by themselves

Cleansing agents

- <u>Soaps, detergents, astringents</u>

  o These remove surface lipids only and not the lipids contained in the pilosebaceous follicle, lipids that are a contributing factor in the pathogenesis of acne

  o Cleansers that contain benzoyl peroxide or salicylic acid have limited efficacy because they are in contact with the skin only during cleansing. They are therefore much less effective than gel or lotion compounds

- <u>Granular or abrasive cleansers</u>

  o Exfoliating action that can aggravate acne by promoting the development of inflammatory lesions

  o To be avoided

- <u>Antiseptic cleansers</u>
  - Contain antiseptics such as triclosan, chlorhexidine
  - Stop surface aerobic bacteria but have no significant effect on *P. acnes*, which are found in the anaerobic environment of the pilosebaceous follicle
- Mild, non-abrasive soaps or cleansers remain the cleansing agents of choice in all cases

Active ingredients

- <u>Benzoyl peroxide</u> (*Benzac AC 5, Benzac W, Benzagel, Clearasil BP, Neostrata, Oxy, Panoxyl, Solugel*)
  - First line of therapy
  - Effective in the treatment of papular lesions
  - Available over the counter in concentrations of 2.5–5%, but no study has shown that efficacy depends on the concentration. Begin with the weakest concentration so as to minimize the skin irritation associated with this product
  - It is recommended that a benzoyl peroxide-based product be applied over the whole treatment area, not just on the lesions
  - Water-based compounds are less drying than alcohol-based ones
  - Water-based gels are less irritating, but acetone- or alcohol-based gels improve the bioavailability of benzoyl peroxide and could therefore be more effective
  - Lotions are less effective than gels, but gels are more irritating
  - **Irritation** is the main side effect, especially among people with fair skin. Irritation is also proportional to the concentration and length of contact time, but tends to diminish over time. Benzoyl peroxide should thus be introduced gradually
  - Other common side effects are dryness of the skin and photosensitivity, for which we suggest using a greaseless sunscreen during the day
  - **Interaction**: benzoyl peroxide can inactivate tretinoin in simultaneous application. If both agents must be used, apply benzoyl peroxide in the morning and tretinoin in the evening

- o Warning: benzoyl peroxide has oxidizing properties and can therefore discolour clothes, bedding, and hair
- o Avoid applying near mucous membranes
- o It may take 6–8 weeks before results can be seen

Table IV: Application of Benzoyl Peroxide-Based Products
Apply for 15 minutes on the first evening and then double the contact time each subsequent evening, up to 4 consecutive hours. After that, the product can be kept on all night.
OR
Apply for 2 hours each evening for 4 evenings, then for 4 hours for 4 evenings, and, after that, all night.
Increase frequency of application up to twice daily.

- Salicylic acid (treatments for acne include *Aveeno*, *Clean & Clear*, *Clearasil*, and *Neutrogena*)
  - o Comedolitic activity, anti-inflammatory
  - o Of controversial effectiveness when the concentration is 2% or less
  - o Must be applied once or twice daily
  - o Has drying properties proportional to concentration
- Sulfur (*Clearasil Acne Control*, *Permox*, *Sulfur Soap*)
  - o Used in concentrations of 2–10%
  - o Frequently associated with salicylic acid or with resorcinol
  - o Of controversial effectiveness
  - o Its colouring helps to hide lesions, but it has an unpleasant odour
- Resorcinol (*Clearasil Acne Control*, *Permox*)
  - o Ineffective when used alone
  - o Can irritate the skin and increase skin sensitivity

When to consult

- If none of these methods are effective after 3 months of use
- If acne is severe, with nodules and/or cysts
- If acne fulminans is suspected due to the appearance of severe acne accompanied by fever and arthralgia
- Possible endocrine etiology (e.g., androgenism, polycystic ovarian syndrome, Cushing's syndrome)
- Large number of lesions
- Intolerance to OTC products

References

- Anonymous. Acne treatment: OTC (non-prescription) [Internet]. Skin therapy Letter. [cited 2007 May 19]. Available from: http://www.skintherapyletter.com/treat/acne/otc.html.
- Bergeron L. L'acné vulgaire. Québec Pharmacie. 1994;41:602-8.
- Caplette A. Le traitement de l'acné vulgaire par des médicaments en vente libre. Québec Pharmacie. 2000;47:505-13.
- Feldman S, Careccia RE, Barham KE, Hancox J. Diagnosis and treatment of acne. Am Fam Physician. 2004;69:2123-36.
- Katsambas AD, Stefanaki C, Cunliffe WJ. Guidelines for treating acne. Clin Dermatol. 2004;22:439-44.
- Klaus D, Placek M, Borelli C, Plewig G. Pathophysiology of acne. JDDG. 2007;4:316-23.
- Mayo Clinic Staff. Acne [Internet]. Mayo Clinic.com: Tools for healthier lives. Mayo Foundation for Medical Education and Research. [cited 2007 May 20]. Available from: http://mayoclinic.com/health/acne/DS00169.
- Purdy S, de Berker D. Acne. BMJ 2006;333:949-53.
- West DP, West LE, Musumeci ML, Micali G. Acne vulgaris. In: Di Piro JT, Talbert RL, Yee GC, Matzke GR, Wells BG, Posey LM, editors. Pharmacotherapy: a pathophysiology approach. 6th edition. United States: McGraw-Hill Companies; 2005. p.1755-68.

Athlete's Foot

Tinea pedis

Overview

- Which organisms are involved?
  - Dermatophytes
  - *Trichophyton rubrum* is the organism most often involved
  - *Trichophyton mentagrophyte* and *Epidermophyton floccosum* are also often present
- Which organisms are involved in a secondary infection?
  - *Candida albicans*
  - *Aspergillus sp.*
  - *Staphylococcus aureus*
  - *Pseudomonas aeruginosa*
- Who is most at risk?
  - More common in men than in women
  - Common among adolescents; uncommon in children
  - More common among active people using public areas (locker rooms and pools)
  - Patients presenting hyperhidrosis
  - Patients with a history of atopic dermatitis
  - Patients with an immune system deficiency (e.g., HIV) or use of immunosuppressive drugs

<u>Questions to ask</u>

✓ **What are the symptoms? (see table below)**

- o Infection is more common in hot and humid climates, and in summer
- o Feet are first to be affected but hands may become infected after
- o Recurrence is common
- o Many types of infection are possible

Table I: Classification of Infection Types			
Types	**Morphology**	**Location**	**Comments**
Interdigital	• Skin fissures, desquamation, and maceration • Often accompanied by pruritus, a burning sensation, and foul odour	• Infection on the side of the toe, especially in the 3rd and 4th spaces Infection can spread to the rest of the foot	• Moisture and heat can exacerbate the condition
Mocassin	• Chronic • Silvery squames on inflamed skin	• Heel, side, and sole of the foot • Toenails often affected • Sometimes affects hands	• Toenails must be treated with an oral agent before any topical treatment of a foot infection
Vesicular	• Less common • Inflamed, vesicular or bulbous lesions • Severe lesions, possible ulceration	• Sole of the foot	• Especially in summer • Mainly caused by *T. mentagrophytes*

What to do

Prevention

- Wear non-occlusive shoes (e.g., sandals) and avoid shoes that are too tight
- Change shoes every 2–3 days to ensure they stay dry
- Wear absorbent cotton socks and change them 1–2 times a day
- After a shower, dry your feet thoroughly, especially between toes
- Do not walk barefoot in public areas (e.g., pools, locker rooms)
- To keep your feet dry, powder inside socks and between toes with talcum powder or medicated powder (e.g., *Tinactin*, *Dr. Scholl's*)
- A thin ribbon of lamb's wool between toes reduces moisture

For an active infection

- Do not share bath towels, socks, or shoes
- Check if family members have been infected
- Wash the affected area with soap and water. Dry thoroughly before applying the antifungal agent
- Do not walk barefoot in the house or in public areas

What to use

- Choose medication with combined antifungal and antibacterial properties, such as clotrimazole or miconazole (imidazole)
- It is recommended to use tolnaftate, undecylenic acid/zinc undecylenate and naftifine for prevention or for adjuvant treatment given the high risk of recurrence and the absence of antibacterial activity. They are often used as aerosols or powders
- Creams are preferred to ointments if the area to be treated is macerated. However, if infection is chronic and marked by dry skin and desquamation, ointment is recommended
- Bid application

- Takes several days–2 weeks to act
- Continue treatment for 2–4 weeks after complete disappearance of symptoms
- <u>Clotrimazole 1%</u> (*Canesten, Clotrimaderm*): **first choice**
  - Acts against dermatophytes and *Candida albicans*
  - Weak antibacterial activity
  - An anti-inflammatory effect has been shown
- <u>Miconazole 2%</u> (*Monistat, Micatin*): **first choice**
  - Antifungal and antibacterial activity
- <u>Tolnaftate 1%</u> (*Tinactin, Dr. Scholl's Athlete's Foot*)
  - Range of action limited to dermatophytes
  - Ineffective against *C. albicans*
  - Higher recurrence compared with treatment with azoles
- Undecylenic acid/zinc undecylenate (*Desenex*)
  - About as effective as tolnaftate
  - Ineffective against *C. albicans*
  - Higher recurrence compared with treatment with azoles
  - Astringent properties of zinc could reduce inflammation and irritation
  - Distinct odour

<u>When to consult</u>

- Patients at high risk of complications, like patients with diabetes and immunosuppression (e.g., HIV or taking immunosuppressive drugs)
- Ungual infection, when topical medication is ineffective
- Evidence of secondary infection (pus-filled lesions, vesicular eruptions, cellulitis)
- Severe inflammation and extremely painful lesions
- No response after 4 weeks of treatment with an OTC agent

References

- Canadian Pharmacists Association. Compendium of nonprescription products. 7th edition. Ottawa: Canadian Pharmacists Association; 2000. p.110-1.
- Gupta AK, et al. Treatments of tinea pedis. Dermatologic Clinics. 2003;21:431-62.
- Habif TP. Superficial fungal infections. In: Hunter J, Savin J, Dahl M, editors. Clinical dermatology. 4th edition. Philadelphia: Mosby Inc.; 2004. p. 409-39.
- Mallin A. Athlete's foot. In: Repchinsky C, Leblanc C, editors. Patient self-care: helping patients make therapeutic choices. 1st edition. Ottawa: Canadian Pharmacists Association; Welcom Ltd: 2002. p. 456-61.
- Potvin C. Quels sont les agents de premier recours pour le traitement du pied d'athlète? Québec Pharmacie. 2002; 49:398-400.
- Pothier D. Le pied d'athlète. Actualité Pharmaceutique. 2004;1-8.
- Weinstein A, Berman B. Topical treatment of common superficial tinea infections. Am Fam Physician. 2002; 65:2095-102.

Burns

Overview

- **Thermal burns**: exposure to flames or to a high-temperature agent (e.g., molten metal, tar, water vapour). Superficial to deep wounds

- **Electrical burns:** usually a deep lesion. Involvement of muscle. Often more serious than they appear. Always consider this kind of wound to be severe, especially when a high-voltage electric current is involved

- **Chemical burns:** exposure to strong acids or to alkaline substances. Alkaline substances are more likely to affect several cutaneous layers

Questions to ask

- ✓ **What agent caused the burn? How did the incident occur?**
- ✓ **How long have you had the burn?**
- ✓ **Where is the burn?**
- ✓ **What is the extent of the burn?**

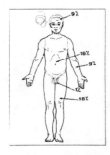

- The burn area can be assessed using the Wallace rule of nines, where the body surface is divided into areas of 9%. This breakdown is not accurate in children. Nevertheless, only a well-trained and experienced professional is able to make a proper assessment of the burned surface area.

✓ **What is the depth of the burn? (see table)**

✓ **How old is the victim?**

✓ **What are the patient's comorbidities?**

Table I: Assessing Depth of Burn			
	Superficial (First-Degree)	**Moderately Severe (Second-Degree)**	**Deep (Third-Degree)**
Tissues involved	Epidermis	Epidermis + dermis	Epidermis + dermis + other tissues
Blisters (phlyctenes)	None	Present	None
Colour	Red	Red	White, charred
Moisture	Dry	Wet	Dry
Sensation	Present	Present	Absent
Pain	Moderate	Intense	Absent
Other	Spontaneous healing	Can be superficial or deep (spontaneous healing impossible)	Spontaneous healing impossible

✓ **What measures have already been taken?**

<u>What to do</u>

First aid

- Remove the cause of the burn
- Cool the affected area as quickly as possible, within 20 minutes of the burn injury
- Flush the burn with cool water (15–20°C) for at least 20 minutes. This procedure also helps to clean the wound of debris. Avoid the use of ice or ice water
- Cover the burn with a loose-fitting, non-adhesive sterile gauze dressing
- <u>Thermal burns</u>
  - o Immerse in cold water (unless there is a very large burned surface area, because there is a risk of developing hypothermia)
  - o Remove any clothing around the burn, but any material adhering to the burn (e.g., nylon or tar) must be left in place
- <u>Chemical burns</u>
  - o If there is any chemical agent present, remove it from the skin
  - o Remove any clothes or jewellry that may have come into contact with chemical substances
  - o Rinse the burn with copious amounts water 15–30 minutes (up to 1–2 hours if it is an alkaline substance)
  - o Check the product label on the chemical substance involved. Call a poison control centre if necessary
  - o A physician must be consulted for burns caused by some chemical substances (e.g., HF, sulfuric acid)
- <u>Electrical burns</u>
  - o Do not touch the victim until you are sure that the voltage source has been eliminated or secured
  - o Remove the voltage source before trying any kind of first aid

- o Send the victim to a physician immediately (emergency): the patient is at risk for cardiac arrhythmia, rhabdomyolysis, and thrombosis
- o While you wait for the ambulance, treat the wound as a thermal burn

Treatment for Burn Healing

- Superficial (first-degree):
  - o Clean with soapy water, 0.9% NaCl or 0.05% chlorhexidine
  - o Apply a moisturizing cream (wait 24–48 hours after the burn to apply)
  - o Protect the wound with dry gauze as needed

- Moderately severe (second-degree superficial):
  - o Clean with soapy water, 0.05% chlorhexidine or ideally, 0.9% NaCl
  - o It is generally not recommended to break the blisters. They should resolve spontaneously in 1–3 weeks, depending on their size. If the liquid inside is not clear (infection is present) or if it is a very large bulla, it could be broken by a physician or a nurse
  - o Debride the wound (can be done with a compress soaked in NaCl or with a jet of NaCl using a syringe
  - o In general, applying antibiotic ointment (e.g., *Polysporin*) is not recommended immediately. It can be considered only if the wound covers a large area or if it shows signs of infection. Application of topical products can make burn assessment more difficult
  - o Dress with porous non-adhesive gauze to protect the wound
  - o Send the patient to a physician if the burn is deep

- Deep burn (second-degree deep or third-degree):
  - o Send the patient to a physician

What to use

- Do not apply the cream immediately. Wait 24–28 hours after the burn incident

- Do not apply any coloured products (e.g., mercurochrome) because these will make wound assessment difficult

- A diluted antiseptic solution of 0.05% chlorhexidine can be used to clean the wound

- Do not put butter or non-sterile fats on the wound

- Do not use topical anaesthetics or topical analgesics, to avoid hypersensitivity reactions

- Use a moisturizing cream to reduce pruritus

- Check the wound daily

- Protect the scar from the sun for 6–12 months after the burn has healed

- Use porous, non-adhesive bandages and gauzes

- <u>Analgesics</u> (see the chapter "Pain"):
  - Acetaminophen (*Tylenol*)
  - Ibuprofen (*Advil*)

- <u>Antibiotic ointment</u>:
  - Not necessary for minor burns
  - Indicated for deep or extensive second-degree burns
  - Keeps the wound moist and avoids the spread of bacteria
  - For oozing wounds, consider cream instead of ointment so as to avoid necrosis
  - Do not damage regenerating tissue with the use of antiseptics (e.g., povidone or chlorhexidine)
  - Bacitracin (*Baciguent*): applied daily before dressing the wound
  - Polymyxin B + bacitracin (*Polysporin*): applied daily before dressing the wound

- Mupirocin (*Bactroban*): applied daily before dressing the wound. Mupirocin is used only when infection or MRSA colonization is suspected or confirmed

When to consult

- Anti-tetanus vaccine necessary (wound is dirty and vaccination history is incomplete or unknown)
- Burns involving young children (< 5 years) and the elderly (> 60 years)
- Deep burns (second-degree deep, third-degree, or charred)
- Second-degree burns involving more than 10% of body surface area in adults and more than 5% in children
- Burns involving the face, genitals, hands, or joints
- Wound healing not progressing (odour, oozing, increasing pain, signs of infection)
- Wound not healed after 2 weeks
- Persistent blistering (sign of a deep burn)
- Signs and symptoms of infection:
  - Redness, heat, and edema around the wound
  - Pus in the blisters or wound
  - Fever, feeling sick
- Electrical burn
- Chemical burn
- Infants with burns
- Inhalation lesions (e.g., patient with facial lesions or stridor, cough, dyspnea, tachypnea)—hospital emergency
- Multiple associated traumas
- Suspected child abuse

References

- Anonymous. Dermatological Emergencies [Internet]. Ottawa: Health Canada; [cited 2007 May 20]: Clinical practice guidelines for nurses in primary care: First Nations and Inuit Health. Available from: http://www.hc-sc.gc.ca/fnih-spni/pubs/nursing-infirm/2000_clin-guide/chap_09_e.html.
- Warren D. Burns. In: Gray J, editor. Therapeutic choices. 3rd edition. Ottawa: Canadian Pharmacists Association; 2000. p.513-19.
- Hartford CE, Kealey GP. Care of outpatient burns. In: Herdon D, editor. Total burn care. 2nd edition. London; WB Saunders. p.40-9.
- Hettiaratchy S, Dziewulski P. ABC of burns: Introduction. BMJ. 2004;328:1366-68.
- Hudspith J, Rayatt S. ABC of burns: First aid and treatment of minor burns. BMJ. 2004;328:1487-89.
- Landry C. Comment traiter un adulte gravement brûlé? Québec Pharmacie. 2005;52:315-26.
- Mayo Clinic Staff. Burn: first aid [Internet]. Mayo Clinic.com: Tools for healthier lives. Mayo Foundation for Medical Education and Research. [cited 2007 May 20]. Available from: http://mayoclinic.com/health/first-aid-burns/FA00022.
- Mayo Clinic Staff. Electrical burn: first aid [Internet]. Mayo Clinic.com: Tools for healthier lives. Mayo Foundation for Medical Education and Research. [cited 2007 May 20]. Available from: http://mayoclinic.com/health/first-aid-electrical-burns/FA000227.
- Mayo Clinic Staff. Burn: first aid [Internet]. Mayo Clinic.com: Tools for healthier lives. Mayo Foundation for Medical Education and Research. [cited 2007 May 20]. Available from: http://mayoclinic.com/health/first-aid-chemical-burns/FA00024.

Chickenpox and Other
Viral Skin Infections

Questions to ask

- ✓ Description and severity of lesions
- ✓ Beginning, frequency, and duration of symptoms
- ✓ Presence of systemic symptoms, including fever
- ✓ Surface area affected and progression
- ✓ Medication history (always suspect drug-induced rash)
- ✓ Treatments and actions till now (efficacy?)

Table I: Characteristics of Various Rashes

Disease	Prodrome	Description of Rash	Incubation Period	Contagious Period and Transmission Mode
Varicella (chickenpox) (*Varicella zoster*)	Fever, malaise, sore throat	1. Macular erythematous rash 2. Vesicles 3. After 2 days, pustules and crusts — Lesions completely healed after 16 days	10–21 days	• 2 days before eruptions, up to 5 days after (crusted lesions = OK) • Transmission via respiratory secretions or contact with lesions
Hand-foot-and-mouth-disease (*Coxsackie* virus A16)	Fever, sore mouth (1–2 days before rash appears)	Grey/white vesicles/ulcers with red halos, in the mouth, on the back, and on the sides of hands and feet (in general), but may affect the palms and soles as well as buttocks; lesions usually asymptomatic. Appears especially during hot months	4–6 days	• From the first appearance of lesions until all vesicles disappear • Transmission via contact with nose and throat secretions, feces
Erythema infectiosum or fifth disease (*Parvovirus* B19)	Fever, malaise, sore throat (arthralgia in adults)	1. Sudden appearance of bright red macular erythematous rash on the face 2. After a day, on the extremities of the extensors and reticular erythema on the trunk with possible duration 7–21 days 3. Recurrence possible due to friction or sun exposure	4–14 days	• Up to 7 days before eruption • Ends when the eruption appears • Transmission via respiratory secretions • From mother to fetus during pregnancy

Table I: Characteristics of Various Rashes

Disease	Prodrome	Description of Rash	Incubation Period	Contagious Period and Transmission Mode
Measles (virus of the *Paramyxovirus* group)	Koplik's spots,[1] fever x 3–4 days, cough, conjunctivitis, coryza	Maculopapular eruptions, first behind ears, then following hairline and spreading downwards, disappearing after 5 days	8–12 days	• 1–2 days before prodrome up to 4 days after rash • Transmission via respiratory secretions
Roseola or exanthem subitum (herpes virus 6 or 7)	High fever 3–4 days	Pink maculopapular rash on neck and especially on the trunk, lasting 1–2 days	7–15 days	• Throughout disease course • Transmission mode unknown
Rubella (German measles) (virus of the *Togavirus* group)	Fever and adenopathy (malaise, sore throat, nauseous and painful occipital lymph nodes in the adult)	Maculopapular erythematous rash starting on the face and neck, then becoming generalized, of short duration (2–3 days))	14–21 days	• 5–7 days before the rash and up to 3–5 days after- Transmission via respiratory secretions • Vertical transmission devastating for the fetus

[1] Greyish pinhead-like points surrounded by a red ring on the buccal mucosa, appearing 24–28 hours before the rash

What to do

Prevention

- Isolation remains the best method, depending on the disease (refer to the table above for contagious periods)

Treatment

- Use an emollient to keep the skin from drying (dry skin exacerbates pruritus)
- Light humidifying of the room
- Good hygiene, non-aggressive cleaning and proper drying of the lesions (dabbing, not rubbing) with mild non-scented soap (choose a syndet bar formulation like *Dove*)
- Be sure to trim fingernails to reduce risk of secondary infection by excessive scratching (children especially)
- Bathe in warm to cold water (pruritus is stimulated by heat, avoid hot baths) 2–3 times per day for 15–20 minutes
- Adding corn starch, sodium bicarbonate, or colloidal oatmeal (*Aveeno*) to the bath can help to reduce pruritus (for maximum effectiveness, be sure to disperse product evenly in the bath)
- Avoid tight clothing, woollen clothing

What to use

Prevention: vaccines

- Varicella: *Varivax III* or *Varilrix*

  o Vaccine with modified live virus. Indicated for everyone aged 12 months and older. Single dose of 0.5 mL SC for children aged 12 months–12 years, 2 doses of 0.5 mL SC at 4–8 weeks apart for adolescents and adults aged 13 years and older. Not recommended to administer booster dose following primary vaccination as described above. Studies show vaccine protects for 14–20 years. Vaccine should not be administered to pregnant women

- Measles: *M-M-R II* or *Priorix*
  - o Vaccine with modified live virus effective against measles, mumps, and rubella (German measles) (MMR), indicated for children over 12 months of age. Two doses at least a month apart are recommended (for children, first dose at 12 months, second dose after 15 months, but before beginning school). Do not administer during pregnancy
- Rubella: *M-M-R II* or *Priorix* (see measles above)
- For a detailed vaccination schedules, see the chapter "Immunization Schedule" in this guide

Treatment

- **Pruritus**
  - o Calamine: Apply on lesions, may dry up skin with prolonged use
  - o Antihistamines: Diphenhydramine (*Benadryl*)
    - – child: 5 mg/kg/day in doses 6–8 hours apart, maximum 300 mg/day
    - – adult: 25–50 mg q6–8h prn
    - – topical preparation not recommended for skin with lesions; be on the lookout for potential allergic sensitization resulting in contact dermatitis
  - o Aluminum acetate solution 0.35% (*Buro-Sol*): Useful against pruritus on damaged skin and on weeping lesions. Soak a gauze pad with solution and apply on the skin for 20 minutes 4–6 times/day; also reduces cutaneous bacterial colonization
  - o Topical corticosteroids: not recommended on weeping lesions, damaged skin, skin presenting a bacterial infection, or for children under 18 months (increased absorption)

- **Fever**
  - Important to properly control body temperature so as to avoid possible complication of febrile convulsions, especially in roseola where fever can be very high
  - <u>Acetylsalicylic acid</u>: not recommended for children with a viral infection due to risk of Reye's syndrome
  - <u>Acetaminophen</u>: child: 10–15 mg/kg/dose q4–6h prn, maximum 65 mg/kg/day OR 5 doses/day; adult: 325–650 mg q4–6h prn, maximum 4000 mg/day
  - <u>Ibuprofen</u>: child: 5–10 mg/kg q6–8h prn, maximum 40 mg/kg/day OR 4 doses/day; adult: 200–400 mg q4–6h, maximum 1200 mg/day

When to consult

- No reduction in pruritus after 48 hours of treatment (especially if the patient scratches continuously, risk of secondary bacterial infection)

- Evidence of secondary bacterial infection

- Fever persists for more than 48 hours under treatment

- Following condition: pregnancy, diabetes, cancer, HIV positive, or chronic consumption of corticosteroids or of immunosuppressors

- Etiology is undetermined

- Viral Infection in an adult (suspect varicella or herpes zoster)

References

- Canadian Pharmacists Association. Compendium of nonprescription products. 41st edition. Ottawa: Association des pharmaciens du Canada; 2006.
- Aoki FY. Herpesvirus infections. In: Gray J, editor. Therapeutic choices. 3rd edition. Ottawa: Canadian Pharmacists Association; 2000. p. 782-7.
- Park KC et Han WS. Viral skin infections: diagnosis and treatment considerations. Drugs. 2002; 62:479-490.
- Tremblay M, Décarie D, Tremblay D; Comité de prévention des infections dans les services de garde à l'enfance du Québec. Les infections en milieu de garde. [Internet]. Quebec. Governemen du Québec. [cited 2007 May 20]. Available from: http://www.mfa.gouv.qc.ca/publications/pdf/SF_aff_infections_milieu_gar de.pdf.
- National Advisory Committee on Immunization. Canadian Immunization Guide, Seventh Edition–2006. Ottawa: Public Health Agency of Canada, p. 374.
- Editorial staff: DiseaseDex®. In: Klasco RK (Ed): DRUGDEX® System. MICROMEDEX, Inc., Greenwood village, Colorado (Edition expires 12/2003). Available from http://www.thomsonhc.com
- Knowles S. Viral skin rashes. In: Repchinsky C, Leblanc C, editors. Patient self-care: helping patients make therapeutic choices. 1st edition. Ottawa: Canadian Pharmacists Association; Welcom Ltd: 2002. p. 573-83.
- Scott LA, Stone MS. Viral exanthems. Dermatol Online J. 2003 Aug; 9: 4.

Corns and Calluses of the Foot
Corns and Calluses of the Foot

Overview

- Corns
  - Lesions caused by thickening of the skin, somewhat elevated, but clearly defined with a yellowish colour
  - Usually located on prominent bony areas (e.g., little toe)
  - Hard Corn: on the lateral side of the little toe or on the dorsal aspect of the toe; dry appearance
  - Soft Corn: between the toes, off-white or yellowish (looks macerated), caused by excessive moisture, very painful

- Calluses
  - Lesions without definite borders, caused by a diffuse thickening of the skin, somewhat elevated and yellowish
  - Usually located in weight-carrying areas, at pressure points (e.g., sole of the feet)

- Differentiate between keratomas and calluses:
  - Keratomas: yellow skin, homogeneous, with round lesions
  - Calluses: in non-sensitive areas, translucent

Questions to ask

- ✓ **Where is the lesion?**
- ✓ **What does it look like?**
- ✓ **Does the patient have any chronic health problems? (Diabetes, circulation problems in your legs, etc.)**
- ✓ **Is the patient taking any drugs regularly? If yes, which ones?**
- ✓ **Any drug-related allergies? (ASA, NSAIDs, etc.)**

- ✓ **When did the problem begin?**
- ✓ **What have you tried?**
- ✓ **What kind of boots or shoes do you wear? Properly fitting? New shoes?**

What to do

- Eliminate the cause of friction or pressure on the feet

  - ○ Avoid narrow and tight-fitting shoes

  - ○ Choose shoes and boots carefully

  - ○ Repetitive use of tools can also cause calluses

- Felt linings, foam, silicon, or moleskin can protect the lesion but won't heal it

  - ○ To protect a corn: the protective pad must surround the lesion

  - ○ Silicone liners can be particularly beneficial for hard corns in that these products release mineral oil, thus enabling a better moisturizing of the lesion

  - ○ To reduce friction (for corns and calluses), the protective liner must be cut to fit the shape and size of the lesion and the area above it

- Soak the foot in warm/hot water for 10–15 minutes a day. With a file or a pumice stone, gently rub the corn and/or callus so as to remove the surface layers of the lesion

- Soften the lesions with a 20% urea-based cream

- To avoid infection, do not use a razor blade or any other sharp cutting edge

- Do not break blisters. Should there be one, treat it with an antibiotic ointment and a dressing

<u>What to use</u>

- Medicated dressings with a salicylic acid base. To be avoided in patients with diabetes or with peripheral vascular disease because such patients require close observation by a specialist

- Available preparations: concentrations from 10–40%:

  o Corn +/- hard or soft: choose weak salicylic acid concentrations (e.g., 12%)

  o Hard corns: choose dressings with high concentrations of salicylic acid rather than plasters or colloids

- Before applying these products, protect healthy skin around the affected area by applying petroleum jelly or nail polish

- Soak the affected area for 10–15 minutes, and then apply the agent for 12–24 hours. Remove whitened skin with a pumice stone. Repeat daily for 6–10 days

Table I: Forms of Salicylic Acid Preparations		
SA Preparations	**Advantages**	**Disadvantages**
Dressing	• Easy to apply • Occlusive/adhesive • Prolonged contact with the lesion	• Trim to the right size, and when applying be careful to avoid healthy skin
Solution	• Occlusive/adhesive	• Be careful during application to avoid healthy skin • The elderly and patients with vision difficulties should avoid this form
Plaster		• The least adhesive and the least occlusive of the 3 forms

When to consult

- Patients with the following conditions:
  - Diabetes
  - Impaired blood circulation in the legs or peripheral vascular disease
  - Foot deformities
  - Serious dermatological problems of the foot
- If the skin is fissured, painful, swollen, or bleeding
- If there is redness around the lesion
- If the patient has a fever
- If the corns and calluses persist despite the treatments
- If there is any abnormal bone structure that is perhaps causing the corns or calluses

References

- Chatlin BE, Barton ED. Corns and calluses [Internet]. eMedicineHealth: Emergency Care+ Consumer Health. [cited 2007 May 19]. Available from: http://www.emedicinehealth.com/corns_and_calluses/article_em.htm.
- Freeman DB. Corns and calluses resulting from mechanical hyperkeratosis. Am Fam Physician. 2002;65:2277-80.
- Goldstein BG, Goldstein AO. Benign neoplasms of the skin [Internet]. UpToDate Online [updated 2007 Mar 15; cited 2007 May 20]. Available from: http://www.utdol.com/utd/content/topic.do?topicKey=pri_derm/7972&type=A&selectedTitle=1~2.
- Mayo Clinic Staff. Corns and Calluses [Internet]. Mayo Clinic.com: Tools for healthier lives. Mayo Foundation for Medical Education and Research. [cited 2007 May 20]. Available from: http://mayoclinic.com/health/corn-and-calluses/DS000033.
- Miller B. Foot care products. In: Carruthers-Czyzewski P, editor. Nonprescription drug reference for health professionals. 1st edition. Ottawa: Canadian Pharmaceutical Association; 1996. p.261-74.

Dandruff

Overview

- Whitish or greyish desquamations in the form of flakes on the scalp, detaching diffusely or in patches

- Sometimes accompanied by pruritus

- Absence of inflammation or erythema

- Precise etiology unknown; possibly caused by the yeast *Pityrosporum ovale*

Questions to ask

✓ **How often do you wash your hair?**

✓ **Does the patient also present with pruritus?**

✓ **Presence of patches?**

✓ **Presence of autoimmune diseases (e.g., psoriasis, HIV, etc.) or use of immunosuppressive drugs?**

What to do

- First of all, suggest washing hair with a mild non-medicated shampoo at least 3 times a week; ideally, every day

- Should a medicated shampoo prove necessary, use it after shampooing with regular shampoo

- UVA and UVB rays inhibit the growth of *P. ovale*. Some exposure to sunshine could reduce symptoms

- If patches are present, before treatment soften these with warm oil (olive oil or mineral oil). Leave the oil on the scalp for several hours or overnight and then wash with a regular shampoo or mild liquid detergent

What to use

*   If regular shampoo is ineffective, **add** a medicated shampoo after shampooing with the regular shampoo

*   Apply shampoo to the scalp and not just to hair

*   Be careful to respect scalp contact time of the medicated shampoo (about 2–5 minutes, depending on the product)

*   Efficacy of medicated shampoos is observed on average after 2–4 weeks

*   In babies, dandruff appears as cradle cap (yellowish detaching crusts). To treat this condition, use a mild shampoo on the scalp, rinsing only after 10–15 minutes so as to soften the crusts. Should that be insufficient, apply baby oil, leaving it on for several hours. In both methods, it is necessary to afterwards remove the crusts with a soft brush. Don't rub too hard. Carry out this procedure once a day. If both methods fail, shampoos with a tar or ketoconazole base of 2% are the alternatives

*   Reassure the parents of the baby, telling them that the condition improves spontaneously at the age of 6–12 months

Table I: Commonly Used Agents in Treating Dandruff		
Agents *Trademarks*	**Directions for Use**	**Precautions and Side Effects**
Antifungal agents		
Ketoconazole 2% *Nizoral*	Treatment: 5–10 mL twice a week for 2–4 weeks Prophylaxis: every 1–2 weeks Contact time: 3–5 minutes	· Greasy/dry hair or scalp · Mild irritation, scalp burning sensation
Zinc pyrithione 1–2% *Head & Shoulders, Dan-Gard*	Apply at least twice a week Can be used daily Contact time: 5 minutes	· Can be used as the only shampoo

Table I: Commonly Used Agents in Treating Dandruff (cont'd)		
Agents *Trademarks*	**Directions for Use**	**Precautions and Side Effects**
Selenium 1–2.5% *Selsun, Selsun Blue, Selegel*	Initially, 5–10 mL twice a week for 2 weeks, then every 1–4 weeks Contact time: 2–3 minutes * Shake well *	· Do not use if there is scalp inflammation · Remove jewellry before using · Every 48 hours only, when used with dye or permanent products · Possible hair loss and seborrhea if used more than twice a week · Possible yellow-orange colouring of grey or white hair. Rinse well after use
Melaleuca (or Tea Tree)	Daily	· Natural product · Controversial efficacy. One study showed that a 5% melaleuca-based shampoo was better than placebo in treating mild to moderate cases when used every day for 4 weeks
Keratolytics: If antifungal products are not effective after 2 weeks or if patches are present, use a keratolytic product		
Coal tar 0.5% (± salicylic acid) *Sebcur/T, Polytar, Tersa-Tar, X-Seb T* *Neutrogena T/Gel*	2–3 times a week as needed or according to manufacturer's directions (especially relieves itching)	· Very irritating, especially in contact with the face · Odour · Can stain skin, hair, clothing · Photosensitivity: avoid exposure to sun for 24 hours after use
Salicylic acid 2–4% *Sebcur, Sebulex, X-Seb*	2–3 times a week	· Irritation · Dryness
Sulfur 2% *Sebulex*	Twice a week	· Irritation · Odour

Table I: Commonly Used Agents in Treating Dandruff (cont'd)		
Agents *Trademarks*	**Directions for Use**	**Precautions and Side Effects**
Antiseptics: Efficacy as sole agent not demonstrated. Often combined with tar		
Triclosan 0.5% *(Tersaseptic)*	Can be used daily	
Povidone iodine 7.5% *(Betadine)*	Apply 10 mL to hair and scalp, and lather with warm water. Rinse and repeat, leaving the lather on the scalp for 5 minutes Treatment: 2–3 times a week for 6–8 weeks Prophylaxis: once a week	• Hypersensitivity to iodine

When to consult

- Severe condition, sudden appearance
- None of these treatments was effective after 2–4 weeks
- Situation worsening
- Presence of an autoimmune disease

References

- American Academy of Family Physicians. Information from your family doctor: seborrheic dermatitis. Am Fam Physician. 2003;68: 1603.
- Canadian Pharmacists Association. Compendium of nonprescription products. 7th edition. Ottawa: Canadian Pharmacists Association, 2000. p.110-1.
- Coupal K. Le traitement de la dermatite séborrhéique et des pellicules. Québec Pharmacie. 2006; 53:437-41.
- Johnson BA. Treatment of seborrheic dermatitis. Am Fam Physician. 2000;61:2703-10.
- Satchell AC. Treatment of dandruff with 5% tea tree oil shampoo. J Am Acad Dermatol. 2002; 47:852-5.
- Sibbald, D. Seborrheic dermatitis, dandruff and psoriasis. In: Repchinsky C, Leblanc C, editors. Patient self-care: helping patients make therapeutic choices. 1st edition. Ottawa: Canadian Pharmacists Association; Welcom Ltd: 2002. p. 508-28.

Frostbite

Frostbite

Overview

- Lesions, superficial or deep, linked to exposure to cold. Such lesions are considered to be burns caused by cold
- Extremities are most often affected: hands, feet, ears, nose
- Frostbite is dangerous and can cause necrosis of the area involved, which may lead to amputation

Questions to ask

✓ **What signs and symptoms does the patient present?**

- o Systemic symptoms (hypothermia)?
  - – Body temperature < 35°C
  - – Shivering and reduced coordination
  - – Possible reduced awareness
  - – Hypotension or hypertension
  - – Tachycardia or bradycardia
  - – Muscular hypertonia, rigidity
- o Local symptoms
  - – (See table below)

✓ **How severe is the frostbite?**

- o On initial evaluation, most frostbitten areas look much alike. Only after warming the affected area can one proceed to a classification of the degree of frostbite severity. (See table below)
- o Determinants of good prognosis:
  - – Normal skin colour
  - – Preservation of tactile sensation
  - – Phlyctenes (blisters) filled with a clear liquid (rather than milky or hemorrhagic)

– Skin is pliable, responding to pressure and then returning to its initial shape

Table I: Evaluation of Frostbite Severity		
	Classification	**Description**
Superficial	First degree	· Central white patch with loss of sensitivity surrounded by an erythematous area · Reversible
Superficial	Second degree	· Phlyctene formation filled with a clear or "milky" liquid in the first 24 hours. Phlyctenes surrounded by edematous and erythematous areas · Reversible but with the likelihood of permanent sensitivity to cold
Deep	Third degree	· Hemorrhagic phlyctene formation resulting in blackish eschars in the 2 weeks after the frostbite
Deep	Fourth degree	· Complete necrosis and loss of tissue · The necrotic tissue may slough off

What to do

First Aid

- Protect the affected area from further trauma

- Begin to warm the affected area only when the patient is in a safe place and when there is no danger of re-exposure to cold. In fact, alternating warming and cooling could exacerbate the lesions. Ideally, warming should be started only once the patient is hospitalized

- Warm the affected area by immersing in water at 40–42°C (the temperature must be accurately measured) for 15–30 minutes or until the skin is warm, flexible, soft, and red. If the skin remains cold and pale, it is probably a deep frostbite. The affected area should be covered with a dry sterile dressing, and a physician must be consulted as quickly as possible

- Avoid rubbing the affected area so as not to exacerbate the lesions

- Dry the affected area, and cover with warm and soft material, without compression

- Immobilize and elevate the affected limb

- Give the patient warm liquids but avoid alcohol or drinks containing caffeine (vasodilation and loss of body heat). Alcohol inhibits shivering and thus diminishes thermoregulatory activity

- If phlyctenes form, leave them alone. Let them break by themselves

What to use

- Analgesics (see the chapter "Pain"):
  - These could be useful to reduce the pain caused by warming the area
  - Acetaminophen (*Tylenol*)
  - Ibuprofen (*Advil*)
    - 400 mg Ibuprofen every 12 hours might limit tissue damage associated with inflammatory mediators (mainly thromboxane A2)

When to consult

- Presence of hypothermia (body temperature < 35°C)

- Deep frostbite or significant superficial frostbite

- Continued loss of sensation after warming

References

- Anonymous. Dermatological Emergencies [Internet]. Ottawa: Health Canada: Clinical practice guidelines for nurses in primary care; First Nations and Inuit Health. [cited 2007 May 20]. Available from: http://www.hc-sc.gc.ca/fnih-spni/pubs/nursing-infirm/2000_clin-guide/chap_09_e.html.
- Biem J, Koehncke N, Classen D, Dosman J. Out of the cold: management of hypothermia and frostbite. CMAJ 2003;168:305-11.
- Foray J. Frostbite. Ann Dermatol Venereol. 2001;128 (10 Pt 1):1075-80.
- McCauley RL, Hing DN, Robson MC, Heggers JP. Frostbite injuries: a rational approach based on pathophysiology. J Trauma. 1983;23:143-7.
- Murphy JV, Banwell PE, Roberts AHN et al. Frostbite: Pathogenesis and treatment. J Trauma. 2000; 48: 171-78.
- White Rowat K. First aid products. In: Carruthers-Czyzewski P, editor. Non-prescription drug reference for health professionals. 1st edition. Ottawa: Canadian Pharmaceutical Association; 1996. p. 223-59.

Fungal Skin Infections

Dermatophytes and tinea versicolor

<u>Overview</u>

- A dermatophyte infection usually causes a circular lesion resulting from an inflammatory reaction that pushes the dermatophyte towards a non-inflamed zone. Thus, the longer the infection lasts, the larger the area of inflammation

- Dermatophytes are classified according to their location on the body

| Table I: Principal Fungal Dermatological Infections ||
Location	Manifestations
Feet *(tinea pedis)*	• The most common fungal infection. (See the chapter "Athlete's Foot")
Body *(tinea corporis or ringworm)* Face *(tinea faciei or incognito)*	• Usually occurs on the trunk and extremities (especially the legs) when the body is affected • Erythematous patch in the form of a circle with an elevated red margin consisting at times of pustules or papules • These are sometimes pruritic and can resemble several other dermatological conditions (e.g., contact dermatitis, erythema multiforme, etc.) • *Tinea gladiatorum* is common among wrestlers
Inguinal region *(tinea cruris)*	• Erythematous patch, at times pruritic, and at times with a margin consisting of pustules or papules • Affects neither the scrotum nor the penis • Caused by heat and humidity (e.g., sweat, wet clothes)
Hands *(tinea manuum)*	• Not common • Same characteristics as on the body (especially on the palms of hands) • Often affects both hands and a foot, or both feet and a hand

Table I: Principal Fungal Dermatological Infections (cont'd)	
Location	**Manifestations**
Beard *(tinea barbae)*	• Especially affects men working with animals • Can be complicated by follicular bacteria or by a pseudofolliculitus
Tinea versicolor or pityriasis versicolor	• Infection caused by the yeast *Malessezia furfur* (and not by a dermatophyte) • Affects areas with sebaceous glands such as the upper trunk, neck, and arms. Can sometimes affect a child's face • Macules or erythematous patches • Affected skin is hypopigmented or hyperpigmented and does not tan • Can sometimes be pruritic • Infection does not resolve spontaneously and can last for years

Questions to ask

✓ **What symptoms have you noticed and how long have you had them? Are the lesions spreading, or have they changed in appearance?**

✓ **Where are the lesions?**

✓ **Have you been in contact with an infected person, animal, or surface?**

   o Dermatophyte infections are contagious

✓ **Do you share personal articles (sandals, running shoes, swimsuits, bath towels)?**

✓ **Do you have lesions on other parts of the body (risk of self-inoculation)?**

What to do

• Know the risk of being infected by others or by animals

• Practice good basic hygiene

• Thoroughly dry your skin after a bath

- Obesity, sedentary lifestyle, and confinement to bed are risk factors for cutaneous mycoses

- Avoid profuse perspiration

- Avoid wearing thick clothes for long periods in hot and humid surroundings

- Choose clothes made of absorbent fabrics (e.g., cotton) and wear loose-fitting undergarments

- Avoid sharing personal articles

- Domestic animals can be transmission vectors. Examine animals for lesions, and take them to a veterinarian if necessary

What to use

- Antifungal creams should be used regularly 1–2 times a day, depending on location

- The product must be applied on the affected area and at least 2 cm beyond its periphery

- Before applying the cream, wash the area and dry it well

- If a cortisone cream must be used at the beginning of the treatment in order to reduce redness and patches, it must be stopped as soon as the symptoms disappear. Topical antifungal treatments must be continued after the symptoms have been resolved so as to prevent re-occurrence

Table II: Topical Treatments		
Location	**Agents Used**	**Application/Duration of Treatment**
Body (*tinea corporis* or ringworm) Face (*tinea faciei* or *incognito*)	· Miconazole 2% bid · Clotrimazole 1% bid	· Up to 1–2 weeks after resolution of symptoms · Treatment for a minimum of 2 weeks
Inguinal region (*tinea cruris*)	· Miconazole 2% bid · *Buro-Sol* or Burrow's solution if maceration is present · Clotrimazole 1% bid · Tolnaftate 1% cream, powder aerosol bid	· Up to 1–2 weeks after symptoms have been resolved, minimum 14 days · If the lesion is perspiring, a powder can be used to dry it up (e.g., *Z-Sorb*). However, do not use if inflammation is present
Hands (*tinea manuum*)	· *Lac-Hydrin* 12% lotion bid · Clotrimazole 1% bid	· Often associated with *tinea pedis* · Treat for at least 10 days · High recurrence rate
Head (*tinea capitis*)	Always in combination with oral treatment: · Ketoconazole 2% shampoo, daily · Selenium 2.5% shampoo daily or lotion daily	· During the entire oral treatment (usually up to 2 weeks after curing) · Shampoos must be applied on the scalp and allowed to remain for 5–10 minutes
Beard (*tinea barbae*)	These products can also be used on asymptomatic carriers	· Combine each treatment with regular shaving and cleansing with antibacterial soap

Table II: Topical Treatments (cont'd)		
Location	**Agents Used**	**Application/Duration of Treatment**
Tinea versicolor or pityriasis versicolor	· Zinc pyrithione 1% daily for 2 weeks (e.g., *Head & Shoulders*)	· Apply for 10 minutes on arms, trunk, or legs and then rinse · Leave it on for 5–10 minutes
	· Selenium 2.5% shampoo daily for 10–14 days and then once a month · Selenium 2.5% lotion (e.g., *Versel*) daily for 1 week OR a 1-dose all-night local application to be repeated in 1 week OR 3–5 times a week for 2–4 weeks	· Leave it on for 10 minutes · Should not be applied on genital areas nor on nipples
	· Ketoconazole 2% shampoo daily for 3 days	· Leave it on for 10 minutes
	· Oral treatment will perhaps be necessary	
	· If the area to be treated is extensive, these products can be applied neck to waist at bedtime to be rinsed in the morning, once a week for 1–4 weeks, depending on the severity of the infection · The patient should be told that pigmentation can take several months to resolve		

Table III: Antifungal Pharmaceutical Forms	
Cream	For desquamating, non-oozing lesions
Ointment	For thick, hyperkeratotic lesions
Liquid	For intertriginous sites, hairy areas, or areas that are oozing, perspiring, or are predisposed to maceration
Powder	Less effective for treatment of already existing infections; more effective as an adjunctive or preventive treatment in reducing moisture and maceration

When to consult

- When *tinea capitis* or *tinea barbae* is suspected
- Extensive infection
- If an animal vector is involved, a visit to a veterinary is necessary
- Patient is immunosuppressed or a diabetic

References

- American Academy of Dermatology. Tinea versicolor. [Internet]. Illinois: American Academy of Dermatology . [cited 2007 February 2]. Available from: http://www.aad.org/public/Publications/pamphlets/TineaVersicolor.htm.
- Anonymous. Treatments for skin, nail and hair infections. [Internet].: Skin Therapy Letter. Skin Care Guide. [cited 2007 May 19]. Available from: http://www.skintherapyletter.com/treat/fungal/skin_nail_hair_treat.html.
- Habif TP. Superficial fungal infections. In: Hunter J, Savin J, Dahl M, editors. Clinical dermatology 4th edition. Philadelphia, Pennsylvania: Mosby Inc., 2004. p. 409-439.
- Hainer BL. Dermatophyte infections. Am Fam Physician. 2003; 67: 101-8.
- Hay RJ. Fungal infections. Clinics in Dermatology. 2006;24:201-12.
- Lemire J. Le tinea et les infections fongiques superficielles. Québec Pharmacie. 2004;51:495-99.
- Mayo Clinic Staff. Acne [Internet]. Mayo Clinic.com: Tools for healthier lives. Mayo Foundation for Medical Education and Research. [cited 2007 May 20]. Available from: http://mayoclinic.com/health/acne/DS00169.
- Vander Straten MR, Hossain MA, Ghannoum MA. Cutaneous infections: dermatophytosis, onychomycosis and tinea versicolor. Infect Dis Clin N Am. 2003;17:87-112.
- Weinstein A, Berman B. Topical treatment of common superficial tinea infections. Am Fam Physician. 2002; 65:2095-102.

Insect Stings and Bites

Insect Stings and Bites

Questions to ask

✓ **Which insect?**
  - *Hymnoptera*: bees, wasps, red ants
  - *Araneae*/spiders: black widow, etc.
  - *Arthropoda* that bite: mosquitoes, black flies, mites, ticks

✓ **Where and when did the incident occur?**
  - Forest, near a lake, flower garden, urban area
  - Any nests around?
  - Day or night?
    - Answers can help to identify the causal agent
    - Almost all systemic reactions occur within 1 hour

✓ **Allergies prior to the insect bite or sting?**
  - Local or systemic reaction

✓ **Patient's current medications**
  - Beware of β-blockers: systemic reaction more severe and often resistance to epinephrine therapy

✓ **Extent of the reaction**
  - Local reaction: surface area helps to grade severity → localized vs extensive, several bites or stings, more than one insect?

✓ **Signs and symptoms?**
  - Local: induration, swelling, redness, pain, pruritus
  - Systemic: generalized itching, flushing, sneezing, watery eyes, nausea, vomiting, muscular cramps, dizziness, fainting, breathing difficulty, arrythmias, hypotension

✓ **Extent of the reaction**

✓ **Signs and symptoms?**

✓ **Products or actions already employed? Efficacy?**

What to do

Prevention

- If possible, avoid situations where you might encounter stinging or biting insects
- Avoid walking in tall grass, stay on paths and walkways
- Avoid using scented cosmetic products
- Avoid wearing brightly coloured clothing (especially white and blue)
- Eliminate stagnant water sources close to the house (birdbaths, basins, etc.)
- Expose minimum body surface
- Use physical barriers such as mosquito netting, pants, and long-sleeved shirts
- Daily inspection for ticks hidden in clothes or already attached to skin, paying close attention to hairy areas, hair, skin folds, neck; remove ticks attached to skin as quickly as possible (within 24 hours) to limit the risk of transmission of Lyme disease or Rocky Mountain spotted fever

Treatment

- Clean the area with soap and water to minimize the risk of secondary infection
- Application of cold compresses (ice in a towel, applied maximum 15 minutes to avoid freezing), reduces pain and swelling while limiting by vasoconstriction the spread of irritant molecules
- Remove stinger, if any, as quickly as possible, with fingernail or credit card
- In the case of red ant bites, do no break pustules (they are sterile) for this risks secondary infection

What to use

Prevention

- <u>DEET</u> (N,N-diethyl-3-methylbenzamide)
  - o Useful against biting arthropods but ineffective against stinging hymnoptera
  - o Can be applied on skin or on clothing
    - – Do not apply on irritated or burned skin nor on an open wound
    - – After use, wash skin with soap and water
    - – When using vaporizer for clothing, avoid vapours for there is risk of neurotoxicity. Use only in well-ventilated areas
    - – Wash clothes after use
    - – Incompatible with synthetic fabrics
  - o Avoid using paradoxical combinations such as sunscreen and DEET (unlimited application for sunscreen vs limited application for DEET)
    - – DEET can decrease the effectiveness of sunscreen
    - – Apply sunscreen 30–60 minutes before applying DEET
  - o Do not use on infants under 6 months; choose physical barriers (clothing, mosquito netting)
  - o Children 6 months–2 years: no vaporizers, use products with concentration of 10% or less, maximum once daily, preferably on clothes
  - o Children 2–12: same as for children 6 months–2 years, but maximum 3 times daily
  - o Adults: 10–30%. Products containing concentration > 30% have been banned in Canada since 2004
  - o Similar efficacy for all concentrations; however, duration of effect is proportional to concentration used (5%, about 2 hours' protection; 15%, about 5 hours' protection)
  - o Pregnant or nursing: use if nonpharmacological methods fail, 10% or less, preferably on clothes only

- P-menthane-3.8-diol (*OFF!* Botanicals)
  - Lemon eucalyptus derivative
  - Protects against mosquito bites for 2 hours
  - Do not use on children under 3 years of age
- Permethrin
  - Useful against biting arthropods, best choice for repelling ticks
  - Can be used on clothes, tents, camping equipment
  - Prolonged effect (~2 weeks)
  - Avoid direct use on skin (highly irritating)
- Citronella
  - Efficacy and protection time less than DEET
  - Do not use on infants under 2 years of age
  - Active protection 30 minutes–2 hours
- Soybean oil
  - Active protection 1–3.5 hours
- Lavender oil
  - Active protection < 30 minutes
  - Do not use on infants under 2 years of age

Treatment

- Calamine lotion
  - Apply on stings to reduce itching
- Oral antihistamines: Diphenhydramine
  - Use to reduce pruritus and swelling
  - Children: 5 mg/kg/day in doses divided q6–8h, maximum 300 mg/day
  - Adults: 25–50 mg q6–8h prn
  - Category B for pregnancy, no data for nursing mothers

- Topical antihistamines: Diphenhydramine
  - Not recommended
  - High risk of allergic sensitization
  - Application up to 4 times daily on healthy skin
  - Avoid prolonged use (> 7 days)
- Topical anesthetics
  - Avoid benzocaine and tetracaine: high risk of allergic sensitization, increased allergy risk with PABA derivatives, sulfonamides, and then by parenteral anesthetics
  - **Pramoxine 1%**: best choice, apply on healthy skin up to 4 times daily
  - **Lidocaine**: less risk of allergic sensitization, apply on healthy skin up to 5 times daily
- Topical corticosteroids: 0.5% hydrocortisone
  - Can help to reduce pruritus, swelling, redness
  - Apply up to 4 times daily maximum 7 days
  - Be alert to risk of bacterial secondary infection
  - Efficacy of preparations < 2.5% limited to reactions mediated by histamine

When to consult

- Signs and systemic symptoms suggesting anaphylaxis (administer epinephrine (*EpiPen*, *Twinject*) IM imperative, high risk of mortality and complications without immediate therapy, administer *EpiPen* 0.01 mg/kg (max 0.3 mg per dose for children and 0.5 mg per dose for adults) q15–20min prn until a medical team arrives)
- Signs and symptoms suggesting a bacterial secondary infection
- No response to treatment
- Increased area of reaction

References

- Covington TR, et al. Nonprescription drug therapy: guiding patient self-care; 2nd edition. St-Louis: Facts & Comparisons; 2003. p. 207-17.
- Freeman TM. Hypersensitivity to hymenoptera stings. N Eng J Med. 2004; 351:978-84.
- Hymenoptera stings. In: POISINDEX® System [Internet database]. Greenwood Village, Colo: Thomson Micromedex. [cited 2007 May 20]. Available from: http://www.thomsonhc.com.
- Lord MC. Problèmes estivaux chez les jeunes enfants. Cahier de FC de l'Actualité Pharmaceutique. April 2007:1-4.
- Pest Management Regulatory Agency. Mosquito Control: Safety Tips on Using Personal Insect Repellents [Internet]. Health Canada. [cited 2007 May 7]. Available from: http://www.pmra-arla.gc.ca/english/consum/insectrepellents-e.html.
- Steen CJ, Carbonaro PA, Schwartz RA. Arthropods in dermatology. J Am Acad Dermatol. 2004; 50: 819-42.
- Wright D. First aid treatment of skin conditions. In: Repchinsky C, Leblanc C, editors. Patient self-care: helping patients make therapeutic choices. 1st edition. Ottawa: Canadian Pharmacists Association; Welcom Ltd: 2002. p. 622-46.

Pruritus

Pruritus

Questions to ask

- ✓ Where is the itch?
- ✓ Are there other symptoms, like difficulty breathing, fever, nausea, and vomiting?
- ✓ How long have you had this condition? Have your lesions become more extensive or have they changed?
- ✓ Is the patient taking a new drug, a new natural product, or new vitamins?
- ✓ Has there been a change in diet?
- ✓ Has there been recent contact with a new substance (e.g., soap, dye, insecticides) or an irritant (e.g., metal, latex)?
- ✓ Is the patient suffering from an illness or a health problem (liver or renal failure, lymphadenopathy, etc.)?
- ✓ Any food or medication allergies?

What to do

- Ensure that the patient does not have dry skin or that he or she does not present other conditions that might cause itching (sunburn, scabies, psoriasis, eczema, dermatophytosis, urticaria, uremia, etc.)

- Check to make sure the reaction is not a side effect of a drug (e.g., an antibiotic) or food

- Try to identify the agent causing the pruritus by elimination:

  o Alcohol, caffeine, and hot drinks can be contributing causes of pruritus

  o Carefully rinse off soap after a shower or bath. Avoid frequent use of soap

- o Suggest that the patient wear light-weight garments, preferably cotton. Avoid wool or other rough clothing
- o Avoid vasodilating substances (spicy foods, caffeine, alcohol, hot water) and profuse sweating
- o Avoid abrupt changes in ambient temperature
- Suggest 20 minutes of warm water compresses, 4–6 times a day
- Suggest sodium bicarbonate baths (125 mL or ½ cup), or colloidal oatmeal (*Aveeno*) or *Buro-Sol*
- Apply a moisturizing cream immediately after a shower
- Should there be a problem of chronic dermatitis, for daily hygiene use a cleanser without soap
- Avoid scratching in order to prevent the appearance of lesions and the risk of infection and scarring

What to use

- Unscented moisturizing lotions
- Phenol- or menthol-based lotions such as the antipruritic lotion *Aveeno* or calamine lotion. A capsaicin-based lotion can also be useful, but its use could be limited by the irritation it causes at the beginning of the treatment. Camphor- or menthol-based substances can decrease sensitivity of nerve endings
- To reduce redness or inflammation, suggest a weak corticosteroid lotion such as *Cortate* (hydrocortisone) 0.5%, 3–4 times a day for a short period of time (maximum of 7 days)
- Calamine has antipruritic properties and can be applied as needed
- If necessary, add an oral antihistamine such as *Benadryl* (diphenhydramine) 25–50 mg for 4–6 hours. Second-generation antihistamines, such as loratadine, desloratadine, and cetirizine can also be used and cause less sedation
- Topical diphenhydramine (e.g., *Caladryl*) is not often recommended because of the risk of contact dermatitis and allergic reaction

- Topical anaesthetics (e.g., pramoxime, benzocaine) are not often recommended because of the risk of allergic reaction
- If the pruritus is located in areas that are often moist (groin, between the toes, under the breasts), suspect a fungal infection and suggest an antifungal cream such as clotrimazole (*Canesten*)

When to consult

- If none of the above suggestions is effective
- No improvement after 7–14 days
- Presence of cutaneous eruptions, large lesions, blisters, ulcers, or fever
- No causal agents found, and continuing pruritus
- Pruritus caused by dermatological conditions (e.g., parasites, psoriasis, lichen planus, eczema) or by systemic conditions (e.g., uremia, cholestasis, celiac disease, HIV, scarlet fever, chickenpox)

References

- Cheigh NH. Dermatologic drug reactions, self-treatable skin disorders, and skin cancer. In: Di Piro JT, Talbert RL, Yee GC, Matzke GR, Wells BG, Posey LM, editors. Pharmacotherapy: a pathophysiology approach. 6th edition. United States: McGraw-Hill Companies; 2005. p.1741-53.
- Fazio SB. Pruritus [Internet]. UpToDate Online [cited 2007 May 19] Available from: http://www.utdol.com/utd/content/topic.do?topicKey=genr_med/35767&type=A&selectedTitle=1~87.
- Katelaris CH, Peake JP. Allergy and the skin: eczema and chronic urticaria. MJA. 2006;185:517-22.
- Lovell O, Vender RB. Management and Treatment of Pruritus. [Internet]. Skin Therapy Letter [2007 February, cited 2007 May 19]. Available from: http://www.skintherapyletter.com/2007/12.1/1.html.
- Mayo Clinic Staff. Itchy skin. [Internet]. Mayo Clinic.com: Tools for healthier lives. Mayo Foundation for Medical Education and Research. [cited 2007 May 20]. Available from: http://mayoclinic.com/health/itchy-skin/DS009847 (Page consluted May 20, 2007).
- Moses S. Pruritis. Am Fam Physician 2003; 68:1135-42,1145-6.
- Wright DE. Dermatitis, seborrhea, dandruff and dry skin products. In: Carruthers-Czyzewski P, editor. Non-prescription drug reference for health professionals. 1st edition. Ottawa: Canadian Pharmaceutical Association; 1996. p. 121-148.

Sun Protection
Sun Protection

Questions to ask

- ✓ **For whom? (children, infants, pregnant women, etc.)**
- ✓ **Is the patient taking any medication? If so, what kind? (Beware of photosensitizing drugs, see Table II)**
- ✓ **Skin type?**
- ✓ **Type of exposure? Short/prolonged? Type of outdoor activity?**
- ✓ **Part of the body exposed?**

What to do

- Limit sun exposure
- Minimize sun exposure 10:00–16:00
- Wear clothes that offer protection: long-sleeved shirt, wide-brimmed hat, pants, and sunglasses that block UVA and UVB rays
- Avoid tanning salons
- Stay in the shade
- Note: all outdoor activities expose skin to UV rays:
  - ○ Up to 90% of rays penetrate the clouds
  - ○ 40% of rays penetrate water up to a depth of 50 cm
  - ○ Snow, ice, sand, and metal reflect up to 85% of UVB rays

What to use

Table I: Types of Sun Filters		
Types	**Examples**	**Characteristics**
Physical filters (or screens)	• Titanium dioxide • Zinc oxide • Talcum powder • Kaolin • Ferric chloride	• Large particles that reflect or diffuse UVA and UVB rays • Opaque • May leave a white film on the skin • Micronized zinc oxide > titanium dioxide
Chemical filters	• Absorb UVA rays (e.g., Parsol 1789) • Absorb UVB rays (e.g., PABA, cinnamates, salicylates) • Absorb UVB and some UVA rays (e.g., benzophenones, anthranilates) • Absorb UVA and UVB rays (e.g., Mexoryl SX)	• Act by absorbing rays • May be combined to obtain a wide-spectrum product • Some have photostabilizing properties (e.g., cinnamates, Mexoryl SX)

- Sun protection factor (SPF)
  - Measures the effectiveness of sun filters against UVB rays only
  - Relationship between the time required to cause the beginning of erythema on skin protected by a sun filter and the time required to cause an equivalent erythema on unprotected skin
    - SPF 15 blocks 93% of UVB rays
    - SPF 30 blocks 97% of UVB rays
    - SPF 60 blocks 98% of UVB rays
- Choose the strength (SPF) according to skin type, state of health, medication being taken, and intensity of the sun (use high-strength products at high altitude)
- Apply sunscreen 30 minutes before exposure; repeat every 2–3 hours or after swimming or heavy perspiration
- Be sure to apply a generous amount of sunscreen

- Sunscreen is not recommended for infants < 6 months. Dress them in protective clothing and keep them in the shade. Do not forget vulnerable areas such as neck and ears
- For babies > 6 months:
  o Sunscreen with an SPF of at least 15
  o Apply sunscreen 30 minutes before exposure, then q2h or after swimming
  o Sunscreen containing PABA is not recommended (associated with contact dermatitis)
  o Choose alcohol-free products
- Pregnant women:
  o Avoid sun exposure, which can result in chloasma
  o Use sunscreen with a high SPF
- Choice of SPF:
  o <u>Agent with an SPF of 15</u>: Patients without special needs
  o <u>Agent with an SPF of 30</u>: Patients with risk factors:
    – Potentially photosensitizing medication
    – Disease exacerbated by UV rays
    – Exposure to the sun in the tropics or at high altitude
  o <u>Agent with SPF of 60</u>: Patients with risk factors:
    – Allergic to UV rays
    – Cutaneous carcinoma
    – Patients who have exhibited a photoallergic or a phototoxic reaction to a medication but who must continue to take it

When to consult

- Characteristics of a lesion that may indicate a melanoma (ABCDE):
  o **A**symmetry
  o **B**order irregularity
  o **C**olour that is not uniform (e.g., beige, brown, black, red, white, blue)
  o **D**iameter greater than 6 mm
  o **E**volution (changes)

Table II: Agents Possibly Causing Photosensitive Reactions		
NSAIDs	**Antineoplastics**	**Diuretics**
Diclofenac	Dacarbazine *	Acetazolamide
Ketoprofen	Fluorouracil	Amiloride
Nabumetone	Methotrexate	Chlorthalidone
Naproxen	Procarbazine	Furosemide
Phenylbutazone	Vinblastine	Indapamide
Sulindac		Metolazone
		Thiazide *
Antibiotics		Triamterene
Azithromycin	**Antipsychotics**	
Tetracycline *	Haloperidol	**CNS drugs**
Quinolones	Loxapine	Carbamazepine
Sulfonamides *	Phenothiazine	Selegiline
	Chlorpromazine	Diazepam
Antidepressants	**Cardiovascular agents**	**Other agents**
Doxepin	Amiodarone	5-ASA
Isocarboxazide	Diltiazem	Auranofine
Maprotiline	Disopyramide	Benzocaine
Paroxetine	Felodipine	Chlorhexidine
Trazodone	Flecainide	Tar derivatives
Tricyclics	Fluvastatin	Sulfonylurea
	ACEIs	Terconazole
	Metoprolol	Tretinoids *
Antihistamines	Nifedipine	Omeprazole
Cyproheptadine	Pravastatin	Quinine
Diphenhydramine	Sotalol	Estrogens
	Terazosine	Progesterone

*Most likely to cause reactions
This is a non-exhaustive list

References

- American Academy of Dermatology. ABCDs of melanoma detection. [Internet]. American Academy of Dermatology. [cited 2007 May 20]. Available from: http://www.aad.org/public/News/DermInfo/DInfoABCDsMelanoma.htm.
- Canadian Dermatology Association. Sun Safe Play, Everyday! [Internet]. Ottawa: Canadian Dermatology Association. [cited 2007 May 7]. Available from: http://www.dermatology.ca/english/newsite/graphics_en/parent_eng.pdf.
- Knowles SR. Reactions relief. What pharmacists need to know about drug-induced skin reactions. Pharmacy Practice. 2004; 20: 38-45.
- Kullavanijaya P, Lim HW. Photoprotection. J Am Acad Dermatol. 2005; 52:937-58.
- Lamoureux J, Dionne A. Les filtres solaires. Québec Pharmacie. 2000; 47:830-7.
- Moore DE. Drug-induced cutaneous photosensitivity. Incidence, mechanism, prevention and management. Drug Saf. 2002; 25:345-72.
- Pellatt S. Sunscreen and tanning products. In: Carruthers-Czyzewski P, editor. Non-prescription drug reference for health professionals. 1st edition. Ottawa: Canadian Pharmaceutical Association; 1996. p. 623-642.
- Robinson JK, Rademaker AW. Sun protection by families at the beach. Arch Pediatr Adolesc. Med 1998; 152:466-70.
- Health Canada. Sunscreens. [Internet]. Health Canada. [cited 2007 May 20]. Available from: http://www.hc-sc.gc.ca/iyh-vsv/life-vie/sun_soleil_e.html.
- Wright D. Cosmetic dermatology. In: Repchinsky C, Leblanc C, editors. Patient self-care: helping patients make therapeutic choices. 1st edition. Ottawa: Canadian Pharmacists Association; Welcom Ltd: 2002. p. 546-72.

Sunburn

Sunburn

Questions to ask

✓ How old is the person?

✓ What areas of the body are involved?

✓ What are the local and systemic symptoms?

✓ When did the sunburn occur?

✓ Is the patient taking photosensitive or phototoxic drugs?
  (See table in the chapter "Sun Protection")

What to do

- Sunburns are the most common first-degree burns, and they are treated in the same way as first-degree burns

- Minor burns:

  o Apply lukewarm water compresses on the affected areas for 20 minutes or soak the affected area in cold water

  o Apply moisturizing cream or lotion on the burn. (Wait 24–48 hours after exposure)

  o Aloe-vera-based products can be used to reduce pain

  o Avoid sun exposure until skin has healed completely Damaged skin is at risk of burning again

  o Make sure the patient is well hydrated because exposure to the sun increases loss of body water

- A minor burn can heal in a few days or, depending on extent and depth, take as much as 3 weeks to heal

- Preventive measures: Because of the complications related to repeated sunburn (e.g., aging of the skin, actinic keratosis, skin cancer), preventive measures are called for, and these should be taken not only for direct sun but also under cloudy skies and in winter. Snow reflects 80% of UV radiation)

  o Minimize sun exposure 10 am–2 pm, when UV radiation is most intense

  o Cover up with clothes and hats

  o Use a sunscreen. (See the chapter "Sun Protection")

  o Wear sunglasses that block 99% of UV rays and that cover a wide field of vision

What to use

- Moisturizing lotion to prevent and to treat skin dryness and desquamation

- Acetaminophen or ibuprofen to relieve pain. For dosage, refer to the chapter "Pain"

- Avoid vaporizers and anaesthetic ointments (risk of allergic reaction)

- Use a sunscreen

When to consult

- Infant < 2 years or the elderly

- Severe burn with blistering

- Sunburn of the eye

- Burns over a wide area of the body surface (risk of systemic involvement)

- Burns accompanied by systemic symptoms (headache, fever, shivering, nausea, vomiting)

- Presence of atypical lesions (e.g., changes in pigmented moles and new nevi)

References

- Goldstein B, Goldstein AO. Diagnosis and management of malignant melanoma. Am Fam Physician. 2001;63:1359-68.
- Laviolette M, Meunier P. Les brûlures mineures. Québec Pharmacie. 2002;49:221-224.
- Mayo Clinic Staff. Sunburn: first aid [Internet]. Mayo Clinic.com: Tools for healthier lives. Mayo Foundation for Medical Education and Research. [cited 2007 May 20]. Available from: http://mayoclinic.com/health/first-aid-sunburn/FA00028.
- Mayo Clinic Staff. Sunburn. [Internet]. Mayo Clinic.com: Tools for healthier lives. Mayo Foundation for Medical Education and Research. [cited 2007 May 20]. Available from: http://mayoclinic.com/health/sunburn/DS00964.
- Pellatt SG. Sunscreen and tanning products. In: Carruthers-Czyzewski P, editor. Non-prescription drug reference for health professionals. 1st edition. Ottawa: Canadian Pharmaceutical Association; 1996. p. 623-642.

Warts

Verruca vulgaris

Overview

- Hyperkeratotic circular lesions of viral origin, with presence of capillaries in their deep portion

- Lesions are well defined, greyish in colour, and surrounded by hyperkeratinized tissue. They can also be black as a result of thrombosed capillaries

- Warts are an infection caused by the human papilloma virus (HPV) The most common infection is found on the plantar aspect of the foot. There are numerous types of HPV infections, the main ones being types 1 and 2

- Type 1 HPV presents isolated lesions described as solitary. Such lesions are deep and painful

- Type 2 HPV is characterized by a less painful mosaic cluster of lesions requiring slightly longer treatment due to their extensiveness

- HPV is highly contagious

Questions to ask

✓ **Visiting public areas?**
  - gyms
  - pools
  - locker rooms
  - physician's offices

✓ **Sharing personal items?**
  - sandals
  - running shoes
  - bathing suits
  - bath towels

✓ **Any lesions present on other areas of the body? (risk of self-inoculation)**

✓ **What are the perceived symptoms, and how long have they been present?**

  o Typically, lesions are found on areas of bony prominence (85%) and on pressure points

  o Also found on traumatized areas (e.g., bitten fingernails)

  o Pain

What to do

- There is no treatment for eradicating HPV

- Without treatment, the warts disappear spontaneously in 6 months in 20–30% of cases and within 2 years in 65% of cases. Quite variable in duration, from several weeks to several months to several years to a lifetime

- Therapy aims at accelerating their disappearance

Prevention

- Avoid sharing personal items

- Avoid walking barefoot in public areas

- Use alcohol to clean personal items that have come in direct contact with warts

Treatment

- Keep the affected area dry (e.g., in the case of plantar warts, wear cotton socks)

- Protect the wart from external trauma by means of an adhesive bandage or dressing

<u>What to use</u>

- Apply products after soaking warts in warm water 5–15 minutes so as to increase effectiveness of treatment

- It is not necessary to treat a plantar wart if there is no pain. Explain that often the wart will disappear spontaneously. However, this increases risk of spreading to other parts of the body and to other people

- <u>Salicylic acid 11–40%</u> (e.g., *Duofilm, Compound W, Dr. Scholl's Clear Away, Soluver*)

  o Keratolytic agent

  o Available as liquid, gel, collodion, or discs (medicated patches)

  o Often combined with lactic acid (e.g., *Duofilm liquid, Duoplant*) that increases effectiveness of salicylic acid

  o Use higher concentrations for thicker skin areas (e.g., plantar aspect of the foot)

  o Apply on clean, dry wart until it disappears (about 12 weeks)

  o Application rates vary depending on the product (qd, bid or q48h)

  o Remains the first line of treatment due to proven effectiveness, safety, and no convincing data showing the superiority of any other agent (e.g., cryotherapy)

  o OTC salicylic acid is contraindicated for patients with diabetes, peripheral vascular disease, or neuropathy

Table I: Application of Salicylic Acid-Based Product
1. Soak the affected area in a warm bath 5–10 minutes
2. Rub the lesion gently with a pumice stone or emery file (nail file)
3. Protect healthy skin surrounding the lesion using petroleum jelly or nail polish
4. Apply product on the affected area and then cover with a dressing if product is a liquid or gel
5. Repeat these steps according to manufacturer's directions (qd, bid or q48h depending on the product) until the skin is healthy again (12 weeks maximum)

- Occlusion
  - Occlusion of a wart is current practice; occlusion with a highly adhesive tape (e.g., duct tape or other fabric-type adhesive tape) stimulates an immune response by causing an irritation
  - One study showed this technique to be superior to cryotherapy
  - The technique consists of cutting a piece of white tape or duct tape just large enough to cover the wart, leaving it in place for 6 consecutive days. Then remove tape, soak wart in warm water, and debride with a pumice stone or emery file. Next day, cover it again with tape and repeat operation for a maximum of 2 months until the wart disappears. The tape can be removed for the night, then replaced with new tape the following morning
  - A response should be seen within 2–3 weeks. If no response, stop after 3 weeks

- Cryotherapy (*Compound W Freeze Off, Dr. Scholl's Freeze Away, Wartner*)
  - Mechanism of action based on liquid nitrogen. The liquid freezes the wart and causes necrosis about 10 days following application. However these products freeze the wart at a temperature higher than that of liquid nitrogen as applied by a doctor and consequently may not be as effective
  - These products are recommended for people over 4 years of age
  - It is recommended that these products be used above a bathroom or kitchen sink
  - Not to be used on facial or genital warts
  - Main side effects are tingling sensation, irritation, pain, temporary whitish discolouration of skin. Incorrect use may also cause neuropathy. OTC cryotherapy is contraindicated in patients with diabetes, peripheral vascular disease, or neuropathy

Table II: Cryotherapy at Home
1. Choose an applicator that best matches wart size
2. Place liquid on applicator by putting it on the vaporizer and spraying 2–3 seconds
3. Touch wart with applicator for 10–40 seconds, depending on the product used or area treated. Only warts on hands or feet can be treated at the same time
4. A bulla or blister may form under the wart. The wart should fall off within 10 days. If it does not, repeat in 10–14 days
5. If wart has not fallen off after 3 treatments (10-day intervals), consult a physician

- Cantharidine 0.7% (*Canthacur, Cantharone*)
  - Blistering agent
  - Sold OTC, but must be applied by a physician or podiatrist

When to consult

- Numerous lesions

- Lesions on the face and on genitals

- No improvement after 12 weeks of treatment, or exacerbation of the condition

- Patient is a diabetic or has arterial or venous insufficiency (peripheral vascular disease)

- Patient immunosuppressed

References

- Benz JD. Cryotherapy versus duct tape for treating warts. Pharmacist's Letter 2002;18:181-216.
- Focht DR 3rd, Spicer C, Fairchok MP. The efficacy of duct tape vs. cryotherapy in the treatment of verruca vulgaris (the common wart). Arch Pediatr Adolesc Med. 2002; 156:971-74.
- Gibbs S, Harvey I. Topical treatments for cutaneous warts. Cochrane Database of Systematic Reviews 2006, Issue 3. Art.No.: CD001781.
- Habif TP. Warts, herpes simplex and other viral infections. In: Hunter J, Savin J, Dahl M, editors. Clinical dermatology 4th edition. Philadelphia, Pennsylvania: Mosby Inc., 2004.
- Mallin A. Plantar Warts. In: Repchinsky C, Leblanc C, editors. Patient self-care: helping patients make therapeutic choices. 1st edition. Ottawa: Canadian Pharmacists Association; Welcom Ltd: 2002. p. 468-71.
- Miller B. Foot care products. In: Carruthers-Czyzewski P, editor. Non-prescription drug reference for health professionals. 1st edition. Ottawa: Canadian Pharmaceutical Association; 1996. p. 261-74.
- Saab Y. Le traitement des verrues vulgaires et plantaires. Cahier de FC de l'Actualité pharmaceutique. January 2007;1-4.

Mouthcare

Cold Sores

Herpes labialis

Overview

- Herpes is caused by two viruses: *herpes simplex virus 1* (HSV-1) and *herpes simplex* virus 2 (HSV-2). Type 1 herpes affects mainly the lips or other areas of the face while type 2 affects mainly the genitals. This section will discuss only the type 1 virus

- There are six stages in a cold-sore episode:
  - Prodrome: irritation, tingling, burning in a localized area
  - Erythema
  - Papule/edema
  - Ulcer
  - Crust
  - Healing

- Average duration of an episode is 3–10 days

- Factors possibly favouring recurrence:
  - Stress or intense emotions
  - Hormonal changes (e.g., menstruation)
  - Irritation of the lips
  - Fatigue
  - Sun
  - Fever

- Frequency of recurrence varies depending on the individual and can range from several weeks to several years

- After primary infection, the virus remains latent in the organism, possibly giving rise to future outbreaks of labial herpes

Questions to ask

- ✓ Is this the first episode?
- ✓ What are the perceived symptoms and how long have they been present?
- ✓ What factors may have caused recurrence?

What to do

- Prevent recurrence due to sun exposure: apply a lip balm that includes a sunscreen
- During prodrome (first 24 hours), ice application could reduce risk of cold-sore appearance
  - o Anecdotal: no study has demonstrated this effect
- Avoid scratching or touching lesions to reduce risk of spreading
- Avoid eye rubbing (the cornea is an ideal site for spreading the virus)
- Avoid close contact with infants and with ill or immunocompromised persons

What to use

- **Systemic analgesics**
  - o Acetaminophen and ibuprofen can relieve pain. Ibuprofen has the advantage of controlling inflammation as well. Especially useful during primary infection
- **Topical analgesics**
  - o Several products are on the market:
    - – *Anbesol*
    - – *Zilactin*
    - – *Viractin*
  - o These products contain various concentrations of benzocaine (5–20%) or lidocaine for pain relief
  - o Short active period (5–10 minutes)

- o Apply as needed
- o Warning: prolonged use may cause sensitivity to local anesthetics and eventual allergic reactions

- **Heparin sodium (*Lipactin*)**
  - o Efficacy more or less documented
  - o Apply on lesions 5 times/day until healed

- **Docosanol 10% (*Abreva*)**
  - o Inhibits virus penetration and therefore cell replication
  - o Reduces infection period by about 18 hours compared with placebo
  - o Must be applied 5 times/day from beginning of prodromal symptoms, for 4 days

- **L-lysine**
  - o Amino acid that inhibits replication of HSV
  - o Oral supplementation
    - 2–3 grams/day for acute treatment, starting when first prodromal symptoms appear
    - 1 gram/day as prevention
    - Side effects: diarrhea and abdominal pain
  - o Topical application (*Lysine +*): applied q2h

- All creams must be applied gently on the affected area, without rubbing, so as to avoid spreading the virus and to reduce risk of physical trauma that may prolong healing time

- **Aluminum acetate 0.35% (*Buro-Sol*)**
  - o Helps to relieve tingling or burning sensation
  - o Apply as needed for 10 minutes or so, 3–4 times/day

- **Emollients**
  - o Apply on dry lesions (crusts)
  - o Help to prevent cracking or fissuring of lip

Warning: Avoid use of:

- o Caustic substances (phenol/silver nitrate)
- o Products containing zinc as an astringent
- o Topical corticosteroids (hydrocortisone)
- o Alcohol

When to consult

- Pregnant woman, nursing infant, immunocompromised patient
- Patient with systemic symptoms
- Disseminated lesions
- Symptoms not relieved by nonpharmacological methods or by OTC products
- Frequent recurrence

References

- Jellin JM, Gregory PJ, Batz F, Hitchens, K, et al. Pharmacist Letter/Prescribers' letter natural medicines comprehensive database. 7th edition. Stockton, CA: Therapeutic Research Faculty; 2005: 825-6.
- MacCara ME. Cold sores. In: Repchinsky C, Leblanc C, editors. Patient self-care: helping patients make therapeutic choices. 1st edition. Ottawa: Canadian Pharmacists Association; Welcom Ltd: 2002. p. 786-92.
- Repchinsky C, Welbanks L, Bisson R, Dang T, Fortin K, Jovaisas B, et al. Compendium of self-care products: the Canadian reference to OTCs. Ottawa: Canadian Pharmacists Association; 2002:3:156-7.
- Sacks SL, Thisted RA, Jones TM, Barbarash RA, Mikolich DJ, Ruoff GE, et al. Clinical efficacy of topical docosanol 10% cream for herpes simplex labialis: A multicenter, randomized, placebo-controlled trial. J Am Acad Dermatol. 2001; 45:222-30.
- Siegel MA. Diagnosis and management of recurrent herpes simplex infections. JADA. 2002; 133:1245-9.
- Sims KM. Oral pain and discomfort. In: Berardi RR, et al., editors. Handbook of nonprescription drugs: an interactive approach to self-care. 13th edition. Washington: American Pharmaceutical Association; 2002. p. 647-76.
- Sing BB, Udani J, Vinjamury SP, Der-Martirosian C, Ghandi S, Khorsan R, et al. Safety and effectiveness of an L-lysine, zinc, and herbal-based product on treatment of facial and circumoral herpes. Alternative medicine review. 2005;10:123-27.
- Spotswood LS and Kriesel JD. Treatment of herpes simplex labialis. Herpes. 2002; 9:64-69.

Dentin Hypersensitivity

Overview

- Sudden pain caused by various stimuli when these come in contact with exposed dentin
- Causes of dentin hypersensitivity:
  o Abrasion (e.g., vigorous brushing, objects in the mouth)
  o Attrition (e.g., bruxism, clenching of teeth)
  o Erosion (e.g., gastrointestinal reflux, eating acidic foods)
  o Gingival recession (loss of gingiva covering the roots of teeth)

Questions to ask

✓ **What are the symptoms?**
  o Sharp pain, short duration, caused by various stimuli:
    – Chemical stimuli (e.g., acidic foods)
    – Thermal stimuli (e.g., hot or cold foods)
    – Mechanical stimuli (e.g., brushing teeth)
    – Osmotic stimuli (e.g., sweet foods)

✓ **Are there special health problems or a special dental condition (e.g., gastric reflux, repeated vomiting)?**

✓ **What has been used till now?**

✓ **Have dental products like tooth whitening kits been used?**

  o Such products notably provoke temporary dentin hypersensitivity that disappears after several hours, but can last several months in some individuals with more fragile dentition

What to do

- Determine the triggering factors
- Reduce consumption of acidic foods (e.g., citrus fruit, carbonated soft drinks)
- Avoid brushing teeth too vigorously or too often

What to use

- **Toothpastes**
  - Strontium chloride (e.g., *Sensodyne*):
    - occlusion of dentinal tubules
  - Potassium nitrate (e.g., *Sensodyne-F*), *Crest Sensitivity Protection Toothpaste*, *Aquafresh Sensitive*):
    - Desensitizes nerves, which results in reduced pain signal transmission to the brain
    - Should prove more effective than strontium chloride
- Use: brush teeth with these agents regularly twice a day
- May take 2–4 weeks of treatment to be effective

When to consult

- Persistent pain despite using medicated toothpastes for 4 weeks

References

- Bourassa, M. Dental conditions. In: Repchinsky C, Leblanc C, editors. Patient self-care: helping patients make therapeutic choices. 1st edition. Ottawa: Canadian Pharmacists Association; Welcom Ltd: 2002. p. 770-75.
- The Canadian advisory board on dentine hypersensitivity. Consensus-based recommendations for the diagnosis and management of dentin hypersensitivity. J Can Dent Assoc 2003; 69: 221-6.
- Orchardson R, Gillam DG. Managing dentin hypersensitivity. JADA. 2006;137:990-8.
- Poulsen S, Errboe M, Lescay Mevil Y, Glenny AM. Potassium containing toothpastes for dentine hypersensitivity. The Cochrane Library 2007; 2:1-15.

Halitosis

Bad Breath

Overview

- Bad breath can be related to:
  - Poor oral hygiene: dental plaque, tooth decay, gingivitis, dry mouth, denture maintenance
  - Food: garlic, alcohol, onions
  - Medications: lithium salts, penicillamine, griseofulvin, thiocarbonate
  - Systemic causes: diabetic ketoacidosis, liver failure, hepatic cirrhosis, uremia, pulmonary abscess
  - Airway disorders: sinusitis, tonsillitis, rhinitis
  - Gastrointestinal disorders: gastroesophageal reflux

What to do

- Identify and eliminate the underlying cause

- Maintain good oral hygiene
  - Brush and floss regularly
  - Scrape the tongue to eliminate bacteria and food particles on the back of the tongue. Several studies show that this is the most effective method for reducing bad breath
  - Tongue must be scraped as far back as possible because bacteria are usually found back 10 cm or more from the tip of the tongue

- Stop smoking

- Chew sugar-free gum (to keep mucosa moist)

- Drink lots of water

What to use

- Use mouthwash or an essential-oil-based gargle (e.g., *Listerine*) or a 0.3% triclosan-based gargle (not available in Canada)

  o Avoid alcohol because it can exacerbate the problem (according to the American Dental Association's Council on Dental Therapeutics)

  o Use mouthwash at bedtime because contact will be longer. As well, bacterial activity causing bad breath is greater at night

- Use a toothpaste with triclosan (e.g., *Colgate Total*)

When to consult

- Problem persists despite good oral hygiene

References

- Blanchette HM. Les maux de la bouche. Québec Pharmacie. 2001; 48:493-4.
- Carvhalo MD, Tabchoury CM, Cury JA, Toledo S, Nogueira-Filho GR. Impact of mouthrinses on morning bad breath in healthy subjects. J Clin Periodontol. 2004; 31:85-90.
- Farrell S, Somogyi-Mann M, Witt JJ. Oral malodor reduction by a combination of chemotherapeutical and mechanical treatments. Clin Oral Invest. 2006;10:157-63.
- Faveri M, Hayacibara MF, Pupio GC, Cury JA, Tsuzuki C, Hayacibara RM. A cross-over study on the effect of various therapeutic approaches to morning breath odour. J Clin Periodontol. 2006; 33:555-60.
- MacCara ME. Halitosis. In: Repchinsky C, Leblanc C, editors. Patient self-care: helping patients make therapeutic choices. 1st edition. Ottawa: Canadian Pharmacists Association; Welcom Ltd: 2002. p.793-7.
- Pedrazzi V, Sato S, de Mattos MG, Lara EH, Panzeri H. Tongue-cleaning methods: a comparative clinical trial employing a toothbrush and a tongue scraper. J Periodontol. 2004; 75:1009-12.
- Pray WS. Afraid to exhale? Help for halitosis. [Internet]. New York. Medscape. [cited 2005 January 17]. Available from: http://www.medscape.com/viewarticle/407619. Quirynen M.
- Management of oral malador. J of Clin Periodontol. 2003; 30:17-8.
- Repchinsky C, Welbanks L, Bisson R, Dang T, Fortin K, Jovaisas B, et al. Compendium of self-care products: the Canadian reference to OTCs. Ottawa: Canadian Pharmacists Association; 2002-3. p. 159.

Oral Ulcers

Aphthous Ulcers

Overview

- Also known as aphthous stomatitis
- Affects 5–25% of general population
- 50% of cases are recurrent within the 3 following months
- Lesions are not contagious
- Symptoms:
  - Burning or tingling sensation about 24 hours before the ulcer appears
  - Painful lesions cause local hypersensitivity and difficulty eating, drinking, swallowing and/or talking
  - Lesions generally disappear in 7–14 days
- **Description**
  - Round or oval lesions 3–10 mm in diameter, covered with a yellowish or grey membrane
  - Contour clearly outlined, surrounded by an erythematous halo
  - Develop on non-keratinized tissues of the mouth
  - 1–5 lesions can be present
- Several factors predispose to appearance of oral ulcers but etiology remains unknown in 80% of cases
  - Stress
  - Hormonal changes (luteal phase of the menstrual cycle)
  - Unbalanced diet (deficiencies in iron, vitamins B_1, B_2, B_6, B_{12}, and C, folate, zinc, or calcium)
  - Chemical products contained in some foods
  - Lesions in the buccal mucosa (bites, burn, injury from hard foods or dental prostheses)

- o Oral colonization by *Streptococcus sanguis*
- o Heredity
- o Allergies (food additives, essential oils, mint, gluten, sodium lauryl sulfate contained in several toothpastes)
- o Inflammatory, autoimmune, or systemic diseases (e.g., fever with pharyngitis or adenitis)
- o Drugs (NSAIDs, barbiturates, beta-blockers, 5-fluorouracil, methotrexate, opioids, phenytoin, salicylates, chemotherapy)
- o Stopping or restarting tobacco use

Questions to ask

- ✓ **Location, number, size, appearance of lesions?**
- ✓ **How long has patient had them?**
- ✓ **History and frequency of lesions?**
- ✓ **Any predisposing factors present?**
- ✓ **Pain intensity and general discomfort?**

What to do

- **Goals:** Control pain and discomfort. Promote healing
- Identify and eliminate predisposing factors
- Avoid foods that cause pain (citrus fruit, sour/acidic substances, tomatoes, chocolate, salt, spices, alcohol, vinegar, melons, and strawberries) or that cause lesions (nuts, hard candy, crackers, and chips)
- Apply ice to lesions
- Maintain good oral hygiene (brush teeth twice a day [soft toothbrush] and floss once a day)
- Eat a balanced diet. If the problem is recurrent and a vitamin deficiency is suspected, advise daily dose of a multivitamin or a complex of vitamins B (B_1, B_6, and B_{12})

- Rinse mouth several times/day with warm water, with a saline solution, or a sodium bicarbonate solution to dislodge mucus and food particles

What to use

- **Cleansing agents**
  - <u>Sodium chloride</u>: ½–1tsp per 240 mL warm water
  - <u>Sodium bicarbonate</u>: 1tsp per 120 mL warm water
  - <u>Sodium perborate 68.6%</u> (*Amosan*):
    - 1 pouch (1.7 g) in 30 mL of warm water
    - Use 3–4 times/day
    - Not recommended for children < 6 years
  - <u>Hydrogen peroxide 3%</u>:
    - Apply undiluted solution directly on the lesion using a cotton swab, up to 4 times/day
    - Diluted in the same amount of warm water (1:1)
    - Use 3–4 times/day to maximum of 14 days (can damage teeth)
    - Avoid in children < 2 years
  - No evidence that sodium perborate or hydrogen peroxide are more effective than a saline solution

- **Protective agents**
  - <u>Inert insulating substances</u>:
    - carboxymethylcellulose/carmellose, gelatin, pectin, and glycerine (*Orabase*)
    - hydroxycellulose-based creams (*Zilactin*), adhere longer than *Orabase*
  - Apply locally as needed before eating and at bedtime
  - Temporarily soothes and relieves pain

- **Astringents**
  - Zinc, aluminum, and tannic acid (*Zilactin*)
  - Apply locally
  - Temporary relief of irritation caused by lesions, dries lesions and promotes healing

- **Topical Anesthetics**
  - <u>Benzocaine 5–20%</u> (*Anbesol, Hurricaine, Mandelay, Orajel, Oragard-B, Topex, Ultracare, Zilactin-B*)
  - <u>Lidocaine 2–5%</u> (*Xylocaine Viscous, Zilactin-L*)
  - Apply locally as needed 3–6 times/day before eating and at bedtime
  - Use with analgesics or protectors to prolong relief
  - Duration of action in monotherapy: 20–30 minutes
  - Loss of sensitivity can make deglutition difficult or cause burns with hot food or drinks
  - Available in gel, ointment, or paste form. The gel contains alcohol; its application can cause a burning sensation. Helpful to apply ice before using a gel
  - Combination of the ingredients of some products is of questionable value (Ineffective or unsafe concentrations or products)
  - Avoid products with high camphor, menthol, or phenol content (can irritate the buccal mucosa)
- **Analgesics taken orally** (see the chapter "Pain")
  - <u>Acetaminophen, acetylsalicylic acid, or ibuprofen</u>
  - Do not dissolve an acetylsalicylic acid tablet in the mouth (can cause irritation)
- **Other**
  - <u>Diphenhydramine oral solution</u>
    - Reduces irritation and pain
    - Gargle 2 minutes then expel, or apply locally with a cotton swab, as needed
  - <u>*Maalox* suspension (aluminum and magnesium)</u>
    - Gargle and expel
- **Ineffective Treatments**
  - Oxygenating agents (e.g., carbamide peroxide 10% in glycerine), zinc sulfate po, lactobacillus preparations and antiseptics (benzalkonium, proviodine, gentian violet, tincture of myrrh, etc.)

When to consult

- Presence of whitish lesions in oral cavity or other lesions not matching the description of aphthous ulcers

- Persistent lesions for more than 2 weeks

- Frequent lesions (6–12 times/year)

- Lesions more than 5 in number

- Lesions more than 10 mm in diameter

- Fused lesion blooms forming an irregular lesion

- Uncontrollable pain associated with difficulties in chewing or swallowing

- Other symptoms: fever, cutaneous lesions, eruptions, uveitis, conjunctivitis, genital ulceration, recurrent diarrhea with blood or mucus, adenopathy, or joint pain

References

- Akintoye SO, Greenberg MS. Recurrent aphtous stomatitis. Dental Clin North Am. 2005; 49:31-47.
- Anonymous. Canker scores. In: Covington TR, editor. Non-prescription drug therapy: Guiding patient self-care. 1st edition. St-Louis: Facts and Comparisons; 2002. p. 793-9.
- Blanchette HM. Les maux de la bouche. Québec Pharmacie. 2001; 48: 493-4.
- Jurge S, Kuffer R, Scully C, Porter SR. Recurrent aphtous stomatitis. Oral Dis. 2006;12:1-21.
- MacCara ME. Aphthous ulcers. In: Repchinsky C, Leblanc C, editors. Patient self-care: helping patients make therapeutic choices. 1st edition. Ottawa: Canadian Pharmacists Association; Welcom Ltd: 2002. p. 779-86.
- Repchinsky C, Welbanks L, Bisson R, Dang T, Fortin K, Jovaisas B, et al. Compendium of self-care products: the Canadian reference to OTCs. Ottawa: Canadian Pharmacists Association; 2002-3. p. 156-7.
- Scully C. Aphtous ulceration. N Engl J Med. 2006; 355:165-72.

Thrush
Oral Candidiasis

Overview

- The most usual causal agent is *Candida albicans*, a yeast often present in normal intestinal flora and in the oral cavity, especially in the tongue area

- *Candida* growth can involve several factors:
  - Environmental: maceration, humidity, heat
  - Physiological: pregnancy, infancy, advanced age, diabetes
  - Immune system deficiency: HIV, corticosteroids, antineoplastics, immunosuppressors
  - Drugs: anticholinergics, antidepressants, antipsychotics, antihypertensives, antihistamines, antibiotics, inhaled corticosteroids

- **Description**
  - Thrush presents in the form of whitish patches, sometimes painful, on the buccal mucosa, tongue, and lips

What to do

- Eliminate causal agent, if possible

- Advise maintaining good oral hygiene

- Advise mouth rinsing after each administration of an inhaled corticosteroid, but do not swallow rinse water

- Use a spacer/holding chamber with a metered-dose inhaler

- Avoid sweet foods (e.g., honey, juice) that promote yeast growth

- If nursing or an infant is involved, wash all materials with soap and water after each use (dishwasher is all right) and sterilize daily with boiling water

What to use

- **Clotrimazole** 1% topical cream (*Canesten*)
  - Application in the mouth 4 times/day
  - If nursing, apply after each feeding
- **Clotrimazole** 100 mg vaginal tablet (adults)
  - Suck 1 vaginal tablet 5 times/day for 14 days (do not swallow)
- **Gentian violet** 0.25%–1%
  - Application once a day. **Maximum 3 days**
  - **For refractory cases only,** because it can cause mucosal irritation or ulceration
  - Aesthetically unpleasant (staining of mucosa)
  - Product is available in 1% concentration only. Dilute with sterile water to obtain concentration of 0.25%–1%
- In case of nursing infants, the mother's nipples must be treated with the same agent

When to consult

- Always tell patient to see a physician

References

- MacCara ME. Oral candidiasis. In: Repchinsky C, Leblanc C, editors. Patient self-care: helping patients make therapeutic choices. 1st edition. Ottawa: Canadian Pharmacists Association; Welcom Ltd: 2002. p.798-801.
- Sims KM. Oral pain and discomfort. In: Berardi RR, et al., editors. Handbook of nonprescription drugs: an interactive approach to self-care. 13th edition. Washington: American Pharmaceutical Association; 2002. p. 647-76.
- Blanchette HM. Les maux de la bouche. Québec Pharmacie. 2001; 48: 493-4.
- Carver PL. Invasive fungal infections. In: Dipiro JT, et al, editors. Pharmacotherapy: a pathophysiological approach. 4th edition. Connecticut: Appleton & Lange; 1999. p.1839-88.
- Gonsalves WC, Chi AC, Neville BW. Common oral lesions: Part I. Superficial mucosal lesions. Am Fam Physician. 2007; 75: 501.
- Muzyka B. Oral fungal infections. Dent Clin North Am. 2005; 49: 49-65.
- Koletar, SL, Russel JA, Fass RJ, Plouffe JF. Comparison of oral fluconazole and clotrimazole troches as treatment for oral candidiasis in patients infected with human immunodeficiency virus. Antimicrob Agents Chemother. 1990; 34:2267-8.
- Cuttner J, Troy KM, Funaro L, Brenden R, Bottone EJ. Clotrimazole treatment for prevention of oral candidiasis in patients with acute leukemia undergoing chemotherapy. Am J Med. 1990; 88:10S-14S.

Xerostomia
Dry Mouth

Questions to ask

✓ **What are the symptoms?**
- o Dry mouth
- o Reduced saliva production
- o <u>Long-term complications</u>:
  - – Burning sensation, sore throat, oral ulcers
  - – Cracked lips
  - – Halitosis (bad breath)
  - – Increased risk of tooth decay, gingivitis, *Candida albicans* infections
  - – Dysarthria, dysphagia, dysgeusia

✓ **Medication history (prescription and OTC)?**
- o <u>Examples of drugs that can cause xerostomia</u>: anticholinergics, antihistamines, antipsychotics, tricyclic antidepressants, SSRIs, benzodiazepines

✓ **Presence of any special health problems?**
- o <u>Examples of conditions that can cause xerostomia</u>: Sjögren's syndrome, chemotherapy, head and neck radiotherapy, uncontrolled diabetes, depression, HIV

What to do

- Sip water often throughout the day
- Chew sugar-free gum or suck on sugar-free candy
- Avoid carbonated drinks and drinks containing caffeine and/or alcohol
- Maintain good oral hygiene, brush teeth and floss regularly, consult a dentist regularly

- Stop smoking
- Ensure adequate ambient humidity

<u>What to use</u>

- **Saliva substitutes** (*Mouth Kote*, *Moi-Stir*, *Biotene*)
  - Usually contain mucine and carboxymethylcellulose, which help to moisturize the mouth
  - Addition of lysozyme, lactoferrin and lactoperoxidase to these products has an antimicrobial effect, thereby decreasing the incidence of comorbidities associated with xerostomia
  - Duration of action relatively short
  - Use as often as necessary
- **Sialagogue** (*Sialor*: anetholtrithione)
  - Increases saliva production
  - Mechanism of action: increases availability of muscarinic receptors in the postsynaptic membrane
  - Dosage: 25 mg tid before meals
  - Maximal efficacy after several days of treatment
  - Contraindications: jaundice, cirrhosis, hepatic ducts or common bile duct obstruction
  - Gastrointestinal side effects: softening of feces
- **Mouthwash**
  - Use an alcohol-free mouthwash (such as *Biotene*) because alcohol can exacerbate symptoms of xerostomia
  - Use a mouthwash containing fluoride to prevent tooth decay (e.g., *Oral B Fluorinse* 0.05%)

When to consult

- Difficulty swallowing, eating, or taking medication

- Problem persists despite nonpharmacological measures and saliva substitutes

- Possibility that a drug might be causing the xerostomia

- Possibility of oral candidiasis

References

- Canadian Pharmacists Association. Compendium of Pharmaceuticals and Specialties. 38th edition. Ottawa: Canadian Pharmaceutical Association: 2003
- MacCara ME. Dry mouth. In: Repchinsky C, Leblanc C, editors. Patient self-care: helping patients make therapeutic choices. 1st edition. Ottawa: Canadian Pharmacists Association; Welcom Ltd: 2002. p. 802-07.
- Kroll B. Dry mouth. Pharmacy Practice. 1998;14:72-82.
- Porter SR, Scully C. An update of the etiology and management of xerostomia. Oral Surg Oral Med Oral Pathol Oral Radiol Endod. 2004; 97:28-46.
- Scully C, Felix DH. Oral medicine: Update for the dental practitioner. Dry mouth and disorders of salivation. British Dental Journal. 2005; 199:423-27.
- Nagano T, Takeyama M. Enhancement of salivary secretion and neuropeptide (substance P, α-calcitonin gene-related peptide) levels in saliva by chronic anethole trithione treatment. JPP. 2001; 53: 1697-1702.
- Shahdad SA, Taylor C, Barclay SC, Steen IN, Preshaw PM. A double-blind, crossover study of Biotène Oralbalance and BioXtra systems as salivary substitutes in patients with post-radiotherapy xerostomia. European Journal of cancer care. 2005;14:319-26.
- Tenovuo J. Clinical applications of antimicrobial host proteins lactoperoxidase, lysozyme and lactoferrin in xerostomia: efficacy and safety. Oral Diseases. 2002; 8:23-29.

Gastrointestinal Problems

Constipation

Constipation

Questions to ask

✓ **What are the symptoms?**

    ○ Difficulty evacuating, unable to evacuate

    ○ Abdominal pain, bloating

    ○ Sensation of incomplete evacuation

    ○ Nausea

    ○ Vomiting

✓ **When was the last bowel movement?**

✓ **What is the normal frequency of bowel movements (fewer or more than 3 times/week)?**

✓ **Presence of blood in the stool, rectal pain, fever, small-sized stool (e.g., pen-sized) or nausea and vomiting?**

✓ **Physical inactivity or completely immobile?**

✓ **Medication history (by prescription or OTC)?**

    ○ <u>Examples of medications that can cause constipation</u>: anticholinergics, anticonvulsants, antiparkinsonians, calcium channel blockers, calcium, iron, diuretics, opiates, tricyclic antidepressants

✓ **Any special health problems?**

    ○ <u>Examples of disorders that could cause constipation</u>: diabetes, hypothyroidism, Parkinson's disease, depression, irritable bowel syndrome, colon cancer

What to do

• Diet rich in fibre (25–30 g/day). Increase the amount gradually

    ○ Examples: whole grain cereals, fruit, vegetables

    ○ Prune juice and figs are good laxatives

- o Adequate intake of fluids and mobility necessary with fibre-rich diets so as to avoid constipation

- Drink a lot of fluids (1.5–2 litres of water/day, that is, 6–8 glasses), except in cases of cardiac or renal failure, or any other liquid restrictions

- Exercise

- Follow a routine. Have bowel movement at the same time each day (30 minutes after breakfast)

- Avoid resisting the urge to defecate

What to use

- **Bulking agents**
  - o Safe agents that can be used over the long term
  - o <u>Psyllium</u>
    - ¬ Water retention in stool increases bulk of bowel contents and increases peristalsis
    - − Onset of action: 12–72 hours
    - − It is important to consume a lot of fluids during treatment (risk of intestinal or esophageal obstruction)
    - − Side effects: bloating, flatulence (decrease with progressive increases in dosage)
    - − Possibility of psyllium allergy, although rarely seen
    - − Do not take 2 hours before or after other medications
    - − Contraindicated if intestinal obstruction (presenting with nausea, vomiting, abdominal pain) or restrictions on fluids
    - − <u>Metamucil</u> powder
      - - Dosage: 1 tablespoon (formulation with sugar) or 1 teaspoon (sugar-free formulation) 1–3 times/day, starting with a small dose and increasing it gradually
      - - Dissolve in 250 mL water or cold juice and drink immediately. Recommendation: drink a second glass of fluids immediately

- *Metamucil* capsules
  - Dosage: 2–5 capsules 1–3 times/day with 250 mL fluids. Swallow one capsule at a time. Recommendation: drink a second glass of fluids immediately
- *Metamucil* wafers
  - Dosage: 2 wafers 1–3 times/day with 250 mL fluids

○ Calcium polycarbophil
  - Same specifics as for psyllium (above), but causes less bloating and flatulence
  - *Prodiem* caplets
    - Dosage: 2 caplets as needed up to 4 times/day. Drink a large glass of water or other fluids with each dose

○ Methylcellulose
  - Same specifics as for psyllium (above) but causes less bloating and flatulence
  - *Prodiem* powder
    - Dosage: 1 tablespoon 1–3 times/day. Dissolve in 250 mL cold water

○ Inulin (*Benefiber*)
  - Soluble fibre extracted from chicory root
  - Dissolves completely in water and doesn't thicken
  - Side effects similar to psyllium
  - Dosage: 1–2 teaspoons (3–6 grams of fibre) dissolved in 120–240 mL of water up to 3 times/day. Do not take with carbonated drinks

- **Emollients**

○ Docusate sodium and docusate calcium
  - Surfactant stool softeners
  - Onset of action: 12–72 hours
  - Of controversial efficacy: psyllium probably has a superior emollient effect. To be used mainly as a preventive measure
  - Generally well tolerated but sometimes provoke gastrointestinal cramps and nausea

    – Do not use with mineral oil because emollients can increase its absorption
- Docusate sodium dosage: 100–200 mg qd–bid
- Docusate calcium dosage: 240 mg qd–bid

- **Stimulants**
  - Act directly on the intestinal mucosa
  - Stimulate motility and secretion of water and electrolytes
  - Risk of habituation in cases of prolonged use
  - Recommended in cases of opiate use
  - Side effects: abdominal pain, diarrhea, electrolytic imbalance
  - Contraindicated in case of intestinal obstruction (presenting with nausea, vomiting, abdominal pain)
  - <u>Sennosides (*Senokot, ex-lax*)</u>
    - Onset of action: 6–12 hours
    - Dosage: 1–4 tablets (8.6–34.4 mg) qd or bid (maximum 8 tablets/day)
    - Can cause brownish pigmentation of colon
    - Changes urine colour (pink/red or brown/black)
    - Excreted into breast milk (brown coloration of the milk)
  - <u>Cascara sagrada</u>
    - Weaker than sennosides
    - Onset of action: 6–12 hours
    - Maximum daily dosage: 325 mg
    - Contraindicated for pregnant women because it can provoke uterine contractions
  - <u>Bisacodyl (*Dulcolax, Correctol*)</u>
    - Onset of action:
      - tablet: 6–12 hours
      - suppository: 30 minutes
    - Dosage:
      - tablet: 5–15 mg po qd
      - suppository: 10 mg qd prn

- o Ricin oil
  - Onset of action: 2–6 hours
  - Dosage: 15–50 mL qd
  - Can cause uterine contractions; pregnant women should not use it
  - Rarely used

- **Lubricants**

  - o Mineral oil (*Nujol, Agarol, Lansoyl*)
    - Lubrication and stool softening
    - Onset of action: 6–8 hours
    - Dosage: 15–45 mL qd for patients able to sit or to stand
    - Risk of lipoid pneumonia in case of inhalation. Not to be given in prone position. To be avoided for bedridden patients or patients having difficulty swallowing
    - Do not use with an emollient because it can increase mineral oil absorption
    - Reduces absorption of liposoluble vitamins A, D, E, and K in prolonged use
    - Oil-based enema: 120 mL rectal qd

- **Osmotics**

  - o Saline laxatives
    - Water retention in the bowel by osmotic action
    - Onset of action: 30 minutes–3 hours
    - Not recommended for patients with heart or renal failure
    - Not recommended for prolonged use

  - o Magnesium hydroxide (milk of magnesia)
    - Dosage: 15–30 mL qd–bid
    - Interactions: may reduce absorption of iron, tetracyclines, and quinolones
    - Risk of hypermagnesemia in patients with renal failure
    - Risk of hypokalemia in prolonged use

  - o Magnesium citrate (*Citro-Mag*)
    - Dosage: 75–150 mL qd as laxative, 300 mL as cathartic Drink 250 mL water before and after each dose

- Drink it cold (better tasting)
- Interactions: may reduce absorption of iron, tetracyclines, and quinolones
- Risk of hypermagnesemia in patients with renal failure

o Sodium phosphate (*Fleet Phospho-Soda* oral)
- Dosage: 45 mL as cathartic or 20 mL qd as laxative dissolved in 125 mL (½ cup) water. Drink 250 mL water after. It is preferable to take it on an empty stomach
- Risk of hyperphosphatemia, hypocalcemia, hypernatremia and acidosis for patients with heart or renal failure or for the elderly
- Do not administer to patients with a sodium restriction
- *Fleet* enema (see the chapter "Preparing for a Diagnostic Test or for a Surgical Procedure")

o Lactulose
- Sugars (galactose and fructose) are metabolized to acids by colon bacteria: acidification of colon, water retention, and stool softening
- Onset of action: 24–48 hours
- Dosage: 15–60 mL/day, divided doses
- Side effects: flatulence, abdominal cramps, nausea, diarrhea
- Contraindicated in case of low galactose diet (667 mg lactulose = 147 mg galactose)
- Can be used by diabetics because it is not readily absorbed (2%)

o Polyethylene glycol (PEG) 3350 (*Colyte*, *Golytely*, *Peglyte*)
- Organic polymers are not readily absorbed: osmotic gradient causes water retention in the intestinal lumen
- Onset of action: 2–4 days
- 240–480 mL reconstituted solution or 15 g (1 rounded tablespoon) in 240 mL water once a day
- Side effects: nausea, bloating, cramps, flatulence
- Is comparable to lactulose or has even greater efficacy
- Reconstituted solution remains stable 48 hours at room temperature and 30 days refrigerated

- o <u>Glycerin suppositories</u>
  - – Local irritation and osmotic effect; expels only the rectal ampulla
  - – Begins to act in 15 minutes–1 hour
  - – Dosage: 1 suppository qd–bid prn. Moisten the suppository before insertion

Special situations

- **Pregnancy**
  - o Medications of choice: bulking agents, fibre, and emollients
  - o Stimulants only as a last resort should other agents prove ineffective
  - o Ricin oil and cascara sagrada are CONTRAINDICATED (risk provoking uterine contractions)
- **Children**
  - o See the chapter "Constipation in Children"

When to consult

- Blood in stool
- Fever, abdominal pain, nausea, vomiting
- Small-sized stool (e.g., pen-sized)
- No stool for 7 days or more
- Persistent gastrointestinal symptoms for more than 2 weeks or recurrent symptoms for more than 3 months

References

- Anderson A, Fenton G. A comparison of dietary fiber supplements in the treatment of mild constipation (abstract). The American Journal of Gastroenterology. 2000; 95:2545-6.
- Canadian Pharmacists Association. Compendium of nonprescription products. 38th edition. Ottawa: Canadian Pharmacists Association; 2003.
- Brandt LJ, Prather C, Quigley EMM, Schiller LR, Schoenfeld P, Talley NJ. Systemic review of chronic constipation in North America. Am J of Gastroenterology. 2005; 100:S5-21.
- Bowles-Jordan. J. Constipation. In: Repchinsky C, Leblanc C, editors. Patient self-care: helping patients make therapeutic choices. 1st edition. Ottawa: Canadian Pharmacists Association; Welcom Ltd: 2002. p. 222-37.
- Dosh SA. Evaluation and treatment of constipation. J Fam Pract .2002; 51:555-9.
- Freedman MD, Schwartz HJ, Roby R, Fleisher S. Tolerance and efficacy of polyethylene glycol 3305/electrolyte solution versus placebo in relieving opiate induced constipation: a double-blinded placebo-controlled trial. J Clin Pharmacol. 1997; 37:904-7.
- Lembo A, Camilleri M. Chronic constipation. N Engl J Med. 2003; 349:1360-8.
- McRory JW, Daggy BP, Morel JG, Diersing PS, Miner PB, Robinson M. Psyllium is superior to docusate sodium for treatment of chronic constipation. Aliment Pharmacol Ther. 1998; 12:491-7.
- Talley NJ. Management of chronic constipation. Rev Gastroenterol Disord. 2004; 4:18-24.

Diarrhea

Questions to ask

✓ Since when has diarrhea been present?

✓ Presence of fever (39.5°C)?

✓ Vomiting?

✓ Presence of blood in stool (stool black or red)?

✓ Signs of dehydration (reduced urine volume, thirst, dry mouth, feeling weak)?

✓ Taking medication by prescription or OTC?

   ○ <u>Examples of medications that could cause diarrhea</u>:

      – Antibiotics, laxatives, methformin, colchicine, domperidone, misoprostol

   ○ Taking antibiotics recently: possibility of pseudomembranous colitis (*C. difficile*)

✓ Recent trip (traveller's diarrhea caused by virus, bacteria, or protozoa)?

✓ Ingestion of unusual food in the last few hours?

✓ Special health problems (irritable bowel syndrome, Crohn's disease, diverticulitis, immunosuppression)?

What to do

• Rehydration

   ○ It is important to rehydrate in order to prevent electrolytic disorders and dehydration

   ○ Rehydration solutions should contain significant proportions of sodium, glucose, and other electrolytes

   ○ Do not use fruit juice or carbonated drinks because they contain too much sugar and few electrolytes o Instead, use *Gastrolyte*, *Pedialyte* or a homemade solution (see recipe). For a child who is not vomiting, administer, as needed, q20–30 minutes. In case of vomiting, give 10 mL q10–15 minutes using a spoon, an oral syringe, or a baby bottle

Table I: Recipe for a Rehydration Solution
360 mL of unsweetened orange juice without pulp
600 mL of boiled or bottled water
½ tsp. salt

o <u>For infants</u>: Continue breastfeeding, and give the rehydration solution between feedings. For a bottle-fed infant, continue giving the usual milk preparation, diluting it by half with the rehydration solution

o <u>For children and adults</u>: Stop milk products during the diarrhea episode (controversial recommendation), but continue with solid foods if possible

  – Avoid sweet and fatty foods

  – Choose bananas, carrots, rice, soda crackers, and soups/broths

What to use

- <u>Loperamide</u> (*Imodium*)

  o Reduces stool frequency and production, increases stool density, relieves cramps and fecal incontinence

  o Contraindicated with presence of strong fever or blood in stool. Risk of toxic megacolon for patients presenting with pseudomembranous colitis or acute hemorrhagic proctocolitis

  o Contraindicated for children (up to 2 years) and not recommended for children 2–12 except on the advice of a physician

  o Dosage (children and adults aged 12 or older): 4 mg (2 tablets) immediately, followed by 2 mg after each liquid bowel movement (maximum 16 mg/day, which is 8 tablets)

- <u>Bismuth subsalicylate</u> (*Pepto-Bismol*)
  - ○ Contains salicylates, so to be avoided for patients taking anticoagulants, for children (Reye's syndrome), during pregnancy, or in case of ASA allergy
  - ○ Less effective than loperamide
  - ○ Dosage for treatment: 2 tablets or 30 mL every 30 minutes (maximum 8 doses/day, which is 16 tablets or 240 mL)
  - ○ Dosage for preventing traveller's diarrhea: 2 tablets or 60 mL qid (limit prophylaxis to maximum 3 weeks)
  - ○ Side effects: black tongue and black stool

- <u>Attapulgite</u> (*Kaopectate*)
  - ○ Is not systematically absorbed. Attaches to water in the intestinal lumen, thereby reducing liquid in the stool
  - ○ Loperamide is probably more effective in treating diarrhea, but attapulgite can relieve nausea and associated cramps
  - ○ Not to be given to children under 3 years
  - ○ Dosage: Adult: 1200–1500 mg after each liquid bowel movement (maximum 9 g/day)

- <u>Fibre such as psyllium</u> (*Metamucil, Prodiem*)
  - ○ Use with small amount of fluids (enough to avoid esophageal obstruction)

When to consult

- Presence of fever, severe abdominal pain, profuse diarrhea, significant vomiting, blood in stool, or signs of dehydration
- Persistent diarrhea for more than 48 hours or recurrent for more than 4 weeks
- Possible case of pseudomembranous colitis (recent use of an antibiotic, fever [39.5˚C], greenish and profuse stool and nausea and cramps)
- Infants under 6 months
- Special health problems (irritable bowel syndrome, Crohn's disease, diverticulitis, immunosuppression)

References

- Canadian Pharmacists Association. Compendium of nonprescription products. 38th edition. Ottawa: Canadian Pharmacists Association; 2003.
- Brownlee HJ. Family practitioner's guide to patient self-treatment of acute diarrhea. Am J Med. 1990; 88:27S-29S.
- Dupont HL, Sanchez JF, Ericcson CD, Mendiola Gomez J, Dupont MW, Cruz Luna A, et al. Comparative efficacy of loperamide hydrochloride and bismuth subsalicylate in the management of acute diarrhea. Am J Med. 1990; 88:15S-19S.
- Dupont HL, Ericsson CD, Dupont MW, Cruz Luna A, Mathewson JJ. A randomized, open-label comparison of non-prescription loperamide and attapulgite in the symptomatic treatment of acute diarrhea. Am J Med. 1990; 88:20S-23S.
- Dukes GE. Over-the-counter antidiarrhea medications used for the self-treatment of acute nonspecific diarrhea. Am J Med 1990:88: 24S-26S.
- Ericsson CD, Johnson PC. Safety and efficacy of loperamide. Am J Med. 1990; 88:10S-14S.
- Forrester A. Diarrhea. In: Repchinsky C, Leblanc C, editors. In: Repchinsky C, Leblanc C, editors. Patient self-care: helping patients make therapeutic choices. 1st edition. Ottawa: Canadian Pharmacists Association; Welcom Ltd: 2002. p. 238-51.
- King CK, Glass R, Breese JS et al. Managing acute gastroenteritis among children; oral rehydration, maintenance and nutritional therapy. MMWR. 2003; 52:1-16.
- Limoges AM. La diarrhée aiguë chez l'enfant et les risques de déshydratation. Québec Pharmacie. 1997; 44:749-752.
- Thoua N, Emmanuel A. Treating functional lower gastrointestinal symptoms. Clin Med. 2006; 6: 449-52.
- Wingate D, Phillips SF, Lewis SJ, Malagelada JR, Speelman P, Steffen R, et al. Guidelines for adults on self-medication for the treatment of acute diarrhoea. Alimen Pharmacol Thera. 2001; 15: 773-82.

Dyspepsia

Overview

- Episodic or persistent pain or abdominal discomfort, usually in upper quadrant of the abdomen

- Increases in intensity after meals; can be caused by large meals, food irritants, or alcohol consumption

- Can be caused by a problem of gastric motility, gastric hyperacidity, and/or possibly psychological in origin

- Perhaps a warning sign of an underlying disease or condition (ulcer, gastritis or gastroesophageal reflux, in about 20% of patients having dyspepsia)

- Two subgroups of patients with dyspepsia:

  o **Functional dyspepsia (non-ulcer):** symptoms cannot be attributed to an underlying cause/pathology, symptoms are persistent or recurrent, and dyspepsia is not relieved by bowel movement or with change in frequency or formation of stool (eliminate irritable bowel syndrome)

  o **Gastroesophageal reflux:** (see the chapter "Gastroesophageal Reflux")

Questions to ask

✓ **What are the symptoms?**

  o Epigastric pain or abdominal fullness

  o Postprandial bloating

  o Quick satiation

  o Belching

  o Anorexia

  o Nausea, vomiting

- o Pyrosis; however, patients mainly presenting with gastric burns and regurgitation should be treated as suffering from gastroesophageal reflux

✓ **Irritable bowel syndrome?**

✓ **Frequency and intensity of symptoms (severity)?**

✓ **How long have the symptoms been present?**

✓ **Evaluate patient risk factors for ulcer development:**
  - o Age
  - o History of ulcers
  - o Family history
  - o Stress
  - o Tobacco use
  - o Alcohol
  - o Medications (NSAIDs or ASA)
  - o *Helicobacter pylori*

✓ **Evaluate presence of alarming factors in the patient; if yes, send to a physician**
  - o More than 50 years of age
  - o Discomfort associated with chest pain radiating to the back, neck, jaw, or left shoulder/arm
  - o Persistent vomiting
  - o Melena, hematemesis
  - o Dysphagia or odynophagia
  - o Fatigue or unexplained weight loss

✓ **Is the patient taking medications?**

Table I: Medications Possibly Linked to Dyspepsia
NSAIDs (including COX-2 inhibitors)
Acarbose
Alcohol
Oral antibiotics
Biphosphonates
Codeine
Corticosteroids
Iron
Natural products (e.g., ginkgo biloba, St. John's Wort, saw palmetto, garlic)
Metformin
Orlistat
Potassium chloride
Risedronate
Theophylline

What to do

- Stop smoking and stop alcohol consumption

- Lose weight

- Avoid fatty and spicy foods and other foods that could exacerbate the situation

- Eat smaller meals, more often

- Avoid chocolate and caffeine

- Avoid milk products in large amounts

- Avoid lying down after meals

- Avoid stomach-irritating medications like NSAIDs and ASA

- Avoid problem precipitating or exacerbating factors

<u>What to use</u>

- **There is little evidence for the efficacy of treatments for functional dyspepsia. For patients presenting with minor or intermittent symptoms, an antacid, an H_2-receptor antagonist, or alginic acid could be recommended**

- **Antacids or H_2-receptor antagonists**

    o H_2-receptor antagonists have the advantage that they can be taken bid (compared to qid for the antacids) and that they relieve symptoms for a longer period

Table II: Medications for Dyspepsia

Antacids

Agents	Side Effects	Dosage	Contraindications	Comments
Sodium bicarbonate (*Alka-Seltzer*)	• Fluid retention • Flatulence, abdominal distension, belching • Metabolic alkalosis possible in case of prolonged use and heavy doses	• 10–20 mL or 2–4 tablets after eating or at bedtime, prn	• Hypertension • Heart failure • Renal failure • Edema • Cirrhosis	• High sodium content
Aluminum hydroxide (*Amphojel*)	• Constipation • Hypophosphatemia with heavy doses • Osteomalacia and dementia possible in case of prolonged use with renal failure	• 15–45 mL q3–6h or 1 hour or 3 hours after eating and at bedtime • 5 mL = 320 mg AlOH	• To be avoided in patients with renal failure • To be avoided in patients with history of constipation or intestinal obstruction	• Several interactions with medications (e.g., iron, quinolones, tetracyclines, digoxin)
Calcium carbonate (*Tums*)	• Constipation • Belching • Flatulence • Heavy doses can cause milk-alkali syndrome or hypercalcemia	• Chew 500–1000 mg CaCO₃ prn • (equivalent of 200–400 mg of elemental calcium)		• Longer acid suppression than with sodium bicarbonate • Acid rebound possible

Table II: Medications for Dyspepsia

Antacids (cont'd)

Agents	Side Effects	Dosage	Contraindications	Comments
Magnesium salts *(Philips Milk of Magnesia)*	• Diarrhea • Kidney stones reported with trisilicate salts • Hypermagnesemia possible in case of prolonged use with renal failure	• 5–15 mL with a bit of water, up to qid (solution of 80 mg/mL)	• To be avoided in patients with renal failure	
Aluminum and magnesium hydroxide *(Maalox)*	• Diarrhea/constipation • Osteomalacia and dementia possible in case of prolonged use with renal failure • Hypermagnesemia also possible in patients with renal failure	• 10–20 mL qid Maximum: 80 mL/day • 5 mL = 200 mg MgOH + 200 mg AlOH + 20 mg simethicone	• See the respective agents (aluminum hydroxide and magnesium salts)	• Helps to reduce diarrhea episodes or constipation associated with administration of a single agent
Alginic acid *(Gaviscon)*	• Water retention • Nausea, vomiting • Belching • Flatulence	• 10–20 mL after eating or at bedtime Maximum: 80 mL/day • 5 mL = 250 mg sodium alginate + 100 mg AlOH	• Hypertension • Heart failure • Edema	• High sodium content • Available in association with other antacids

Table II: Medications for Dyspepsia

Agents	Side Effects	Dosage	Contraindications	Comments
H₂-receptor antagonists				
Ranitidine (*Zantac*)	• Headache, nausea, vomiting, diarrhea	• Patients 16 or older, 75–150 mg po prn (maximum 300 mg/day)		• Not to be taken for longer than 2 weeks without medical follow-up
Famotidine (*Pepcid*)	• Headache, dizziness	• Patients 12 years or older, 10–20 mg po prn (maximum 40 mg/day)		• Not to be taken for longer than 2 weeks without medical follow-up

When to consult

- Symptoms persisting for more than 2 weeks despite use of antacids or H_2-receptor antagonists
- Risk of an organic cause (gastric cancer, diabetic gastroparesis, etc.)
- Alarming factors or symptoms
  - Age over 50
  - Dysphagia or odynophagia
  - Nausea, persistent vomiting
  - Melena, hematemesis
  - Discomfort associated with chest pain radiating to the back, neck, jaw, or shoulder/left arm. Suspect angina or acute coronary syndrome
  - Fatigue or unexplained weight loss
- Severe pain

References

- Canadian Medical Association. An evidence-based approach to the management of uninvestigated dyspepsia in the era of *Helicobacter pylori*. CMAJ. 2000;162:S3-S23.
- Conroy RT, Siddiqi B. Dyspepsia. Prim Care Clin Office Pract. 2007; 34:99-108.
- Dickerson LM. Evaluation and management of nonulcer dyspepsia. Am Fam Physician. 2004; 70:107-14.
- Fisher RS, Parkman HP. Management of nonulcer dyspepsia. New Engl J Med. 1998; 339:1376-81.
- Henderson R, Prince VT. Heartburn and dyspepsia. In: American Pharmaceutical Association. Handbook of nonprescription drugs. 14th edition. Washington; 2004. p. 317-48.
- Thomson Peter. Dyspepsia and GERD. In: Repchinsky C, Leblanc C, editors. Patient self-care: helping patients make therapeutic choices. 1st edition. Ottawa: Canadian Pharmacists Association; Welcom Ltd: 2002. p. 256-63.
- Talley NJ. Therapeutic options in nonulcer dyspepsia. J Clin Gastroenterol. 2001; 32:286-93.

Gastroesophageal Reflux

Gastroesophageal Reflux

Overview

- Reflux of gastric contents into the esophagus

- Stomach acid contents can damage the larynx, oropharynx, esophagus, and respiratory system

- Frequency, severity, and duration of symptoms characterize pathological reflux as opposed to reflux normally present in an individual

- Esophagitis is reported in 30% of patients newly diagnosed presenting symptoms of gastroesophageal reflux

Table I: Risk Factors for Gastroesophageal Reflux		
Diet	**Medications**	**Other Factors**
Factors that reduce pressure of the lower esophageal sphincter		
Chocolate, garlic, oinions, mint, fatty foods, alcohol	Anticholinergic agents, α-adrenergic antagonists, β_2-blockers, bisphosphonates, calcium channel blockers, ethanol, diazepam, morphine, nitrates, estrogen, progesterone, prostaglandin, tricyclic antidepressants, theophylline	Tobacco use (nicotine)
Factors that slow gastric emptying		
Foods	**Medications**	
Spicy foods, orange juice, tomato juice, coffee	Bisphosphonates, aspirin, NSAIDs, iron, potassium, quinidine, tetracycline, zidovudine	
Factors that increase intragastric pressure		
Obesity, pregnancy, tight clothing, exercise		
Factors that have a direct irritating effect on gastric mucosa		
Duodenal ulcers, endocrine adenomas, tobacco use, Zollinger-Ellison syndrome		

Questions to ask

✓ **What are the symptoms? Since when?**
  ○ Pyrosis
  ○ Pain possibly radiating to the chest, back, and throat
  ○ Burning sensation
    • Symptoms appear especially after meals and at bedtime
    • Symptoms can be mild or persisting
    • Major symptoms such as dysphagia, odynophagia (pain while swallowing), hypersalivation or regurgitation are also possible
    • Some more atypical symptoms like chest pain mimicking angina may also be present
✓ **Current medications?**
✓ **Tobacco use?**
  ○ In some patients, tobacco use can provoke reflux and intensify symptoms

What to do

• Goals
  ○ Reduce symptom recurrence
  ○ Relieve symptoms
• Avoid risk factors possibly leading to gastroesophageal reflux
• Change lifestyle
  ○ Avoid foods that reduce pressure of the lower esophageal sphincter or that slow gastric emptying
  ○ Avoid large meals
  ○ Avoid exercise after meals
  ○ Avoid lying down after meals (wait at least 3 hours)
  ○ Raise the head of bed 10 cm
  ○ Lie on the left side for sleeping

- o Avoid tight clothing
- o Lose weight
- o Stop smoking

What to use

- Antacids
  - o Very few studies support antacid use in treating reflux, despite their popularity. Because of their relatively brief activity period, about 1.5 hours, frequent use is required in order to repress gastric acid over 24 hours. In additon, doses heavier than those in the treatment of dyspepsia are required in order to treat symptoms of gastroesophageal reflux
  - o In general, suspensions should be preferred to tablets because suspensions are more effective in neutralizing gastric acid. Some patients, however, may have difficulty tolerating the taste of these products
  - o Antacids increase stomach and duodenal pH but do not act on acid secretion
  - o Antacids may alter the pharmacokinetics of other medications taken concomitantly. After taking an antacid, it is recommended the patient wait 2 hours before taking another medication

- H_2-receptor antagonists
  - o They inhibit gastric acid secretion by means of linking with H_2 receptors in the parietal cells of the stomach
  - o Inhibiting action depends on the dosage
  - o Dosages offered OTC reduce the frequency of night waking episodes caused by reflux. Briefly, symptomatic relief is similar to relief by antacids but the effect lasts longer

Table II: Pharmacological Treatments for Gastroesophageal Reflux

Agents	Side Effects	Contraindications	Comments
Antacids (see doses in the chapter "Dyspepsia")			
Sodium bicarbonate *Alka-Seltzer*	• Fluid retention • Flatulence, abdominal distension, belching • Metabolic alkalosis possible in case of prolonged use and heavy doses	• Hypertension • Heart failure • Renal failure • Edema • Cirrhosis • Pregnancy	• High sodium content • Occasional use only
Aluminum hydroxide *Amphojel*	• Constipation • Hypophosphatemia in case of prolonged use with very high doses • Osteomalacia and dementia possible in cases of prolonged use in patients with renal failure	• To be avoided in patients with renal failure • To be avoided in patients with history of constipation or intestinal obstruction	• Several interactions with medications (e.g., iron, quinolones, tetracycline, digoxin)
Calcium carbonate *Tums*	• Constipation • Belching • Flatulence • Heavy doses may cause milk-alkali syndrome or hypercalcemia		• Agent of choice for patients with renal failure • Longer acid suppression than with sodium bicarbonate • Acid rebound possible

	Table II: Pharmacological Treatments for Gastroesophageal Reflux		
Agents	Side Effects	Contraindications	Comments
	Antacids (see doses in the chapter "Dyspepsia") (cont'd)		
Magnesium salts	• Diarrhea • Kidney stones with trisilicate salts	• To be avoided in cases of renal failure	
Phillips' Milk of Magnesia	• Hypermagnesemia possible in cases of prolonged use with renal failure		
Combination aluminum/ magnesium	• Diarrhea/constipation • Osteomalacia and dementia possible in cases of prolonged use in patients with renal failure	• See the respective agents (aluminum hydroxide and magnesium salts)	• Helps to reduce episodes of diarrhea or constipation associated with administration of a single agent
Maalox	• Hypermagnesemia also possible in patients with renal failure		
Alginic acid	• Water retention • Nausea, vomiting	• Hypertension • Heart failure • Edema	• Available in association with other antacids
Gaviscon	• Belching • Flatulence		• High sodium content
	H₂ receptor antagonists		
Ranitidine Zantac	• Headache, nausea, vomiting, diarrhea	• Known hypersensivility to the drug or its ingredients	• Not to be taken for longer than 2 weeks without medical follow-up
Famotidine Pepcid	• Headache, dizziness	• Known hypersensivility to the drug or its ingredients	• Not to be taken for longer than 2 weeks without medical follow-up

<u>When to consult</u>

- **Presence of alarming symptoms in the patient**
  - Age over 50 years
  - Discomfort associated with chest pain radiating to the back, neck, jaw, or shoulder/left arm
  - Persistent vomiting
  - Melena, hematemesis
  - Dysphagia or odynophagia
  - Fatigue or unexplained weight loss (more than 3 kg in 6 months for no particular reason)
  - Severe abdominal pain
  - Persistent pain for more than 2 weeks despite use of antacids or H_2-receptor antagonists
  - Blood in stool
- **Possibility of affecting upper respiratory airways**
  - Chronic cough (for at least 3 weeks), sensation of a lump in the throat, wheezing, hoarse morning voice, laryngitis and hiccups, painful and difficult swallowing, heavy coughing accompanied by bleeding

References

- Canadian Medical Association. An evidence-based approach to the management of uninvestigated dyspepsia in the era of *Helicobacter pylori*. CMAJ. 2000; 162:S3-S23.
- Carruthers-Czyzewski P, editor. Gastroesophageal reflux. In: Nonprescription drug reference for health professionals. 1st edition. Ottawa: Canadian Pharmaceutical Association; 1996. p. 282-85.
- Fisher RS, Parkman HP. Management of nonulcer dyspepsia. New Engl J Med 1998; 339:1376-81.
- Henderson R, Prince VT. Heartburn and dyspepsia. In: American Pharmaceutical Association. Handbook of nonprescription drugs. 14th edition. Washington; 2004. p. 317-49.
- Hunt RH. Importance of pH control in the management of GERD. Arch int med. 1999;159:649-57.
- Katz PO. Optimizing medical therapy for gastroesophageal reflux disease: State of art. Reviews in gastroenterological disorders. 2003; 3:59-69.
- Smtih Candace. Gastroesophageal reflux disease. US Pharmacist. December 1999:77-86.
- Thomson Peter. Dyspepsia and GERD. In: Repchinsky C, Leblanc C, editors. Patient self-care: helping patients make therapeutic choices. 1st edition. Ottawa: Canadian Pharmacists Association; Welcom Ltd; 2002. p. 256-63.

Hemorrhoids
Hemorrhoids

Overview

- Blood vessels located under the anal canal mucosa (internal) and under the epidermis of the perianal region (external hemorrhoids) that swell, protrude, and cause various symptoms

- Several factors are involved in the etiology of hemorrhoids: pregnancy, prolonged sitting or standing, low-fibre diet, constipation, diarrhea, straining to lift heavy objects

Questions to ask

✓ **What are the symptoms?**
  - Hemorrhoids can be internal or external (perianal masses)
  - Possibility of pruritus or anal seepage
  - Pain
  - Possible presence of soft skin tags
  - Discomfort or irritation often present (itching, burning sensation, inflammation)
  - Sensation of having something "coming out" of the rectum
  - Bright red bleeding during defecation
  - Presence of blood on the surface of stool only (not mixed with stool), often visible on toilet paper
  - Sensation of incomplete emptying after a bowel movement

✓ **How long have the symptoms been present?**

✓ **Has the patient been using a product to relieve the symptoms?**

✓ **Any special health problems?**

What to do

- Prevent/treat constipation (see the chapter "Constipation"):
  - Fibre-rich diet (25–30 g/day)
  - Drink a lot of fluids (1.5–2 litres water/day, which is 6–8 glasses), except in cases of heart or renal failure
  - Psyllium (*Metamucil*) or methylcellulose (*Prodiem*)
  - Docusate sodium (*Colace*)
  - Avoid laxative stimulants such as *Senokot*
- Sitz bath (hot water) for 15 minutes 3–4 times/day
- Clean the perianal area with water and soap or use witch hazel pads (*Tucks* Medicated Pads) after each bowel movement
- Avoid straining during defecation
- Avoid sitting on the toilet for more than 5 minutes to reduce straining and reduce pressure on the blood vessels affected
- Avoid lifting heavy objects and severe straining
- In a crisis, take a sitz bath 3–4 times/day. Apply ice bags or cold compresses on the anal area for 10 minutes at a time, 3–4 times/day
- In case of severe pain, try bed rest as long as needed

What to use

- <u>Goal of therapy</u>: Relieve symptoms, keep the anal area clean, and facilitate and regularize bowel movements
- There are numerous products such as creams, oinments, and suppositories. However, suppositories often slip deeply into the rectum, passing beyond the treatment area. For this reason, choose creams and ointments
- Before applying a product and after each bowel movement, clean the area carefully with soap and warm water
- <u>Anti-inflammatories</u>
  - Reduce pruritus and inflammation

- Hydrocortisone 0.5% (the only concentration available OTC)
- Limit use to 1 week so as to reduce risk of mucosal atrophy

- Local anesthetics
  - Relieve pain and pruritus
  - Possible hypersensitivity reaction
    - Pramoxine 1% causes fewer allergic reactions
  - Short-term use seems safe (less than 7 days). Prolonged use increases risk of contact dermatitis
  - Benzocaine 20%: apply up to 6 times/day
  - Dibucaine (*Nupercaincal*): apply morning and evening and after each bowel movement (maximum: 30 g/24 hours)
  - Pramoxine (*Anusol* Plus): apply morning and evening and after each bowel movement

- Astringents
  - Decrease irritation, burning sensation, and pruritus
  - Zinc oxide: apply up to 4–6 times/day after each bowel movement
  - Zinc sulfate (*Anusol, Anuzinc*): apply up to 6 times/day after each bowel movement
  - Witch hazel pads (*Tucks* Medicated Pads, *Preparation H PE*): apply up to 6 times/day after each bowel movement

- Antiseptics
  - Prevent microbial activity
  - Domiphen (*Nupercainal* cream)
  - No more effective than soap and water

- Barriers
  - Physical barrier that reduces irritation and prevents significant water loss
  - Glycerin (*Tucks* Medicated Pads): apply up to 4 times/day
  - Shark liver oil (*Preparation H*): apply morning and evening and after each bowel movement
  - Petroleum jelly: apply up to 4 times/day

- o Zinc oxide: apply up to 4–6 times/day
- o Apply after sitz baths and after each bowel movement
- Vasoconstrictors
  - o Blood vessel constriction reduces tissue inflammation
  - o Ephedrine: apply up to 4 times/day
  - o Naphtazoline: apply morning and evening and after each bowel movement
  - o Phenylephrine (*Preparation H PE*): apply morning and after each bowel movement
  - o Possible systemic absorption
    - – To be avoided in cases of hypertension, hyperthyroidism, cardiovascular disease, diabetes, or benign prostatic hyperplasia (hypertrophy)
- Healing substances
  - o Increase speed of healing
  - o Shark liver oil (*Preparation H*): of controversial efficacy
  - o Bio-Dyne skin respiratory factor (*Preparation H*): insufficient evidence to confirm its efficacy
- Possible use of an analgesic po for pain relief (e.g., acetaminophen, ibuprofen)

When to consult

- Bleeding
- Presence of dark-coloured blood
- Patient under 12 years
- Problem lasting more than 7 days
- Prolapse that remains in external position and that must be repositioned manually
- Patient with Crohn's disease or ulcerative colitis (not to be mistaken for symptoms of disease recurrence)
- Family history of colon cancer

References

- Canadian Pharmacists Association. Compendium of nonprescription products. 38th edition. Ottawa: Canadian Pharmacists Association; 2003.
- Beique L, Roy J. Les lésions hémorroïdales. Québec Pharmacie. 1995; 42:241-6.
- Carruthers-Czyzewski P. Hemorrhoids. In: Repchinsky C, Leblanc C, editors. Patient self-care: helping patients make therapeutic choices. 1st edition. Ottawa: Canadian Pharmacists Association; Welcom Ltd: 2002. p. 287-93.
- Chan J, Berardi RR. Anorectal Disorders. In: American Pharmaceutical Association. Handbook of nonprescription drugs. 14th edition. Washington; 2004. p. 433-55.
- Madoff RD, Fleshman JW. American Gastroenterological Association technical review on the diagnosis and treatment of hemorrhoids. Gastroenterol. 2004;126:1463-73.
- Nisar PJ, Scholefield JH. Managing haemorrhoids. BMJ. 2003; 327: 847-51.
- Anonymous. Assessment of the Gastrointestinal System. [Internet]. Ottawa: Health Canada: Clinical practice guidelines for nurses in primary care; First Nations and Inuit Health. [cited 2007 May 18]. Available from: http://www.hc-sc.gc.ca/fnih-spni/pubs/nursing-infirm/2000_clin-guide/chap_05a_e.html.
- Sause RB. Self-treatment of hemorrhoids. U.S. Pharmacists. 1995; 20:32,34-36,39-40.

Intestinal Gas

Intestinal Gas

Overview

- Multifactorial disorder:
  - Malabsorption
  - Lactose intolerance (dairy products)
  - Foods rich in target fermented carbohydrates (grains, potatoes, pulses, etc.)
  - Fructose (honey), sucrose, sorbitol (foods containing sweeteners, gums, sugar-free candy)
  - Carbonated drinks
  - Fatty foods (reduce motility and cause gas retention)
  - Digestive diseases (e.g., gastric ulcers, reflux, irritable bowel syndrome, Crohn's disease, ulcerative colitis, diverticulitis, constipation)
  - Diabetes, hypothyroidism, constipation, cancer
- Changes in large bowel pH
- Medications: antibiotics, narcotics, acarbose, calcium channel blockers, anticholinergics, orlistat, lactulose

Questions to ask

- ✓ **What are the symptoms?**
  - Belching
  - Dyspepsia
  - Cramps
  - Abdominal discomfort
  - Bloating
  - Flatulence
  - Nausea
- ✓ **Recent changes in eating habits?**
- ✓ **Presence of a digestive pathology?**

<u>What to do</u>

- Change eating habits: avoid or reduce consumption of foods that can cause gas: (e.g., broccoli, cabbage, cauliflower, beans)

- Avoid aerophagia (chewing gum, talking while eating)

- Eat slowly and chew food well

- Increase fibre intake gradually

    o Fibre helps to increase intestinal motility but can also cause gas because it is a substrate for fermentation by bacterial flora

- Increase physical activity (increases intestinal motility)

- Drink sufficient amounts of water (increases intestinal motility)

- Avoid lying down after a meal

- Avoid tight clothes and belts

- Patients presenting lactose (milk product) intolerance should avoid dairy products or should eat them with a lactase supplement

What to use

Table I: Products Used for Treatment of Intestinal Gas

Medications	Indications	Mechanism of Action	Side Effects	Dosage
Simethicone Gas-X Phazyme Ovol	Antiflatulent, gently eliminates gases but does not reduce the total quantity of gas produced Mitigated efficacy	Reduces surface tension of gases formed by mucus	No systemic absorption, hence no side effect documented	80–160 mg po prn after eating and at bedtime (maximum 500 mg/day)
α-Galactosidase Beano	Recommended as prophylactic treatment for gases caused by foods rich in fibre (pulses and vegetables)	Hydrolizes oligosaccharides contained in foods before they are metabolized by bacteria in the colon Enzyme deactivated by heat; not to be put in very hot foods	Warning for diabetics: produces 2–6 g of carbohydrates per 100 g of food Produces galactose: to be avoided by patients having galactosemia	150–450 galactose units with first mouthful of food 1 tablet or 5 drops of Beano per ½ cup of gas-forming foods
Lactase Lacteeze Lactaid	Indicated for lactose-intolerant patients	Hydroxylation of lactose facilitates digestion of milk products and prevents utilization of lactose by the intestinal bacterial flora	Well tolerated Drops can be added to a carton of milk and then refrigerated for 24 hours so as to allow lactase to act	3000–9000 FCC** units of lactase before meals **FCC: Food Chemical Codex

When to consult

- Symptoms lasting more than 1–2 weeks
- New symptoms of flatulence accompanied by moderate or severe abdominal pain, nausea or vomiting, fever, shivering
- Unexplained weight loss
- Change in stool colour
- Blood in the stool
- Presence of abdominal pain and severe constipation for several days (suspect ileus)
- Presence of long-term diabetes, celiac disease, history of gastrointestinal pathology

References

- Ganiats TG, Norcross WA, Halverson AL, et al. Does Beano prevent gas? A double-blind crossover study of oral alpha-galactosidase to treat dietary oligosaccharide intolerance. J Fam Pract. 1994; 39:441-45.
- Meek PD. Intestinal gas. In: American Pharmaceutical Association. Handbook of nonprescription drugs. 14th edition. Washington; 2004. p. 349-65.
- Nguyen P. Le traitement des gaz intestinaux. Québec Pharmacie. 2004; 51:572-76.
- Serra J, Azpiroz F, Malagelada JR. Intestinal gas dynamics and tolerance in humans. Gastroenterology. 1998; 115:542-50.
- Thomson Peter. Gas and cramps. In: Repchinsky C, Leblanc C, editors. Patient self-care: helping patients make therapeutic choices. 1st edition. Ottawa: Canadian Pharmacists Association; Welcom Ltd: 2002. p. 264-68.

Nausea and Vomiting

Nausea and Vomiting

Questions to ask

- ✓ **Patient's age?**
- ✓ **Condition related to motion sickness?**
- ✓ **Patient pregnant?**
- ✓ **Nausea/vomiting related to a specific cause?**
  - ○ Pregnancy, chemotherapy, recent surgery, medications, infection, food
- ✓ **How long has patient had the problem?**
- ✓ **Other symptoms such as abdominal pain, headache, diarrhea, fever, or dehydration?**
- ✓ **Taking any medications (prescription or OTC)?**
  - ○ Examples of drugs that could cause nausea/vomiting: acyclovir, NSAIDs, valproic acid, amiodarone, oral contraceptives, antituberculotics, beta-blockers, calcium channel blockers, carbamazepine, colchicine, digoxin, erythromycin, opiates, phenytoin, sulfamides, sulfonylureas, theophylline
- ✓ **Special health problems?**
  - ○ Examples of disorders that could cause nausea/vomiting: appendicitis, gastroenteritis, gastrointestinal obstruction, irritable bowel syndrome, pancreatitis, vestibular disorders, pyelonephritis, chronic renal failure, psychogenic causes (anorexia, bulimia), migraine

What to do

- • Avoid large meals; try eating small amounts of food more often
- • Avoid fatty foods. Rice, toast, and dry biscuits are foods that are usually well tolerated

- Drink plenty of water
- Use a rehydration solution as needed
- Avoid strong odours
- Seek peaceful surroundings
- Avoid taking unnecessary medications
- For pregnant women, choose nonpharmacological means
- For motion sickness:
  o Sit in front seat of a car
  o Look at a distant fixed point
  o Avoid reading or looking through side windows

<u>What to use</u>

- <u>Dimenhydrinate (*Gravol*)</u>
  o Adults and children over 12 years: 50–100 mg po q4–6h prn/ 50–100 mg ir q6–8h prn (maximum: 400 mg po/day)
  o Children 6–12 years: 25–50 mg po/ir q6–8h prn (maximum: 150 mg po/day)
  o Children 2–5 years: 12.5–25 mg q6–8h prn (maximum: 75 mg po/day)
  o Also for children: 5 mg/kg/day divided q4–6h
  o For motion sickness, take the first dose about 30–60 minutes before departure
  o Side effects: sedation, anticholinergic effects (blurred vision, xerostomia, urinary retention, constipation), confusion, paradoxical reactions possible in children
  o Contraindications: glaucoma, benign prostatic hyperplasia, chronic obstructive pulmonary disease, breastfeeding
- <u>Diphenhydramine (*Benadryl*)</u>
  o Adults and children over 12 years: 25–50 mg po q4–6h prn (maximum: 300 mg po/day)

- o Children 6–12 years: 12.5–25 mg po q4–6h prn (maximum: 150 mg po/day)
- o Children 2–5 years: 6.25 mg q4–6h prn (maximum: 37.5 mg po/day)
- o Also for children: 5 mg/kg/day divided q4–6h
- o Side effects: sedation, anticholinergic effects (blurred vision, xerostomia, urinary retention, constipation), confusion, paradoxical reactions possible in children
- o Contraindications: glaucoma, benign prostatic hyperplasia, chronic obstructive pulmonary disease, breastfeeding

- Meclizine (*Bonamine*)
  - o 25–50 mg po q24h prn, to be taken 1 hour before departure in cases of motion sickness (maximum: 50 mg po/day)
  - o Side effects: drowsiness, anticholinergic effects (blurred vision, xerostomia, urinary retention, constipation)
  - o Contraindications: glaucoma, benign prostatic hyperplasia
  - o Not recommended for children under 12 years

- Promethazine (*Histantil*)
  - o Adults: 12.5–25 mg po/pr q4–6h prn
  - o Children: 6.25–12.5 mg po/pr q24h prn
  - o For motion sickness, take the first dose about 1.5–2 hours before departure
  - o Side effects: drowsiness, blurred vision, cutaneous rash, hypotension, dizziness, akathisia, tremors, pseudoparkinsonism
  - o Contraindications: hypersensitivity to phenothiazines, glaucoma, benign prostatic hyperplasia
  - o Not recommended for children under 2 years because of risk of severe respiratory depression

- Scopolamine (*Transderm-V*)
  - o Apply 1 patch (1 mg) on the hairless area behind the ear q72h prn. Apply the patch at least 4 hours before departure (ideally 12 hours before)

- o Wash hands thoroughly after application and avoid contact with eyes (can cause mydriasis)
- o Side effects: drowsiness, anticholinergic effects (blurred vision, xerostomia, urinary retention, constipation), hallucinations, confusion, disorientation
- o Contraindications: pediatric setting, pregnancy and breastfeeding, glaucoma, benign prostatic hyperplasia, liver or renal failure
- o Drug interactions: sedatives, anticholinergics (synergistic effect)

- <u>Vitamin B6 (pyridoxine)</u>
  - o 25 mg po tid
  - o Effective for morning sickness in pregnant women

When to consult

- Pregnant women can use OTC products and drugs only when recommended by a physician
- Signs of dehydration, significant vomiting, or persistent symptoms
- Patient has suffered cranial trauma
- Patient is receiving chemotherapy or radiotherapy
- Possibility of severe food poisoning that does not resolve in 12 hours
- Severe abdominal pain (in the central or lower abdomen) can indicate appendicitis or gastrointestinal obstruction
- Nausea/vomiting with fever and/or diarrhea
- Blood present in the vomit
- Nausea and vomiting induced by eating disorders such as bulimia or anorexia

References

- 2003 Update of the statement of motion sickness. Pharmacist's letter/Prescriber's letter. 2004; 20:2001-22.
- Canadian Pharmacists Association. In: Repchinsky C, Leblanc C, editors. Patient self-care: helping patients make therapeutic choices. 1st edition. Ottawa: Canadian Pharmacists Association; Welcom Ltd: 2002. p. 306-23.
- Carruthers-Czyzewski P, editor. Nonprescription drug reference for health professionals. 1st edition. Ottawa: Canadian Pharmaceutical Association; 1996.
- Sahakian V, et al. Vitamin B6 is effective therapy for nausea and vomiting of pregnancy: a randomized, double-blind placebo-controlled study. Obstet Gynecol. 1991, 78: 336.
- Shane-McWhorter L, Fermo J. Nausea and vomiting. In: American Pharmaceutical Association: Handbook of nonprescription drugs. 14th edition. Washington; 2004. p. 470-491.
- Taketomo CK, Hodding JH, Kraus DM. Pediatric dosage handbook 11th edition. Hudson: Lex-Comp Inc.

Preparing for a Diagnostic Test
or for a Surgical Procedure

Overview

- A colonoscopy is a procedure used to detect colon cancer and to evaluate various gastrointestinal symptoms and problems such as gastrointestinal bleeding, rectal bleeding, abdominal pain, inflammatory abdominal conditions, and anemia

- A preparation must be used to rapidly empty the colon of stool without causing side effects or changes in the intestinal mucosa

Questions to ask

✓ What kind of procedure?

✓ When will the procedure take place?

✓ Presence of comorbidities such as renal failure?

What to do

- To be ingested the evening before the test: meal consisting only of clear fluids

- Liquids allowed before a test: black coffee, regular tea, fruit juices without pulp, carbonated drinks, water. Milk or cream must be avoided

What to use

Magnesium citrate

- Hyperosmotic solution that causes water absorption in the intestinal lumen in order to increase motility

- *Royvac*
  - o Kit includes a bottle containing 296 mL magnesium citrate (17.46 g), 3 tablets of bisacodyl (5 mg) and a bisacodyl suppository (10 mg)
  - o Schedule:
    - – Noon: liquid meal: clear soup (consommé), plain gelatin, 225 mL fluids
    - – 14:00—drink 225 mL fluids
    - – 17:00—drink oral solution (magnesium citrate); onset of action: 3–6 hours
    - – 18:00—liquid meal: clear soup (consommé), plain gelatin, 225 mL fluids
    - – 20:00—take 3 bisacodyl tablets with a large glass of water
    - – 21:00—225 mL fluids
    - – 22:00—insert suppository and hold it in 10–15 minutes, even if there is urgent need to have a bowel movement
    - – At bedtime: 225 mL fluids
  - o Contraindications: renal failure, intestinal obstruction, abdominal pain, or bleeding
  - o Caution: elderly patients, patients on a low-sodium diet
  - o Side effects: hypermagnesemia, electrolytic imbalance possibly causing convulsions, dizziness, weakness

- *Citro-Mag*
  - o See above for contraindications, warnings, and side effects. Consists of a clear solution consisting of 15 g magnesium citrate in 300 mL
  - o Schedule:
    - – Take 225 mL of clear fluids, then the rest of the bottle of *Citro-Mag*, then 225 mL of clear fluids. Drink a glass of water every hour during the 4–5 hours after taking *Citro-Mag*, according to the regimen and the use of concomitant cathartic agents
    - – Use of cathartic agents such as bisacodyl is recommended so as to increase the laxative effect of magnesium

Polyethylene glycol

- A large-volume, iso-osmotic, non-absorbable electrolytic solution that cleanses the intestinal lumen by means of the cathartic effect following large-volume ingestion

- *Colyte, PegLyte, Golytely*

  - Contain polyethylene glycol 3350 in powder form to be reconstituted with water

  - Osmotic agent that does not cause ion loss or absorption, thereby avoiding electrolytic changes. Agent of choice for patients with renal failure

  - If possible, patient must fast for at least 3 hours before beginning to take the solution

  - Add water up to the filling line for a total 4 litres of solution. Do not add artificial flavouring or other ingredients. Shake well until completely dissolved. To improve taste, solution can be refrigerated

  - Schedule:
    - Drink 240 mL of solution every 10 minutes until evacuated water is clear and free of fecal matter (ingestion of 3–4 litres usually necessary). It is better to drink it all at once than to take little sips
    - After taking the solution, ingestion only of clear fluids is allowed before the test or intervention
    - Onset of action: about 1 hour

  - Contraindications: ileus, gastric retention, gastrointestinal occlusion, colonic perforation, toxic megacolon, severe colitis

  - Precautions: patients at risk for pulmonary aspiration or regurgitation

  - Side effects: nausea, abdominal fullness, and bloating, Mallory-Weiss syndrome, colitis, SIADH, decreased systolic pressure, pulmonary aspiration

  - Stability at room temperature after reconstitution: 48 hours

  - Stability refrigerated after reconstitution: 30 days

  - Modified regimens of polyethylene glycol combined with bisacodyl are better tolerated and do not interfere with efficacy when compared with the standard 4 L dosage regimen (for example, PEG 2 L + bisacodyl 10 mg–20 mg = efficacy similar to PEG 4 L)

Sodium phosphate

- A low-volume hyperosmotic solution that increases water content of intestinal lumen so as to create a cathartic effect

- *Fleet Enema, Fleet Phospho-Soda*
  o Oral solution:
    - Bottle with 45 mL solution (5 mL lemon-ginger flavoured laxative containing 2.4 g sodium phosphate monobasic and 0.9 g sodium phosphate dibasic)
    - As purgative, drink all the solution in the bottle (45 mL)
    - Each 45 mL dose should be taken with at least 240 mL water or clear fluids, followed by an additional 480 mL water or clear fluids
    - Recommended single maximum daily dose of sodium phosphate oral solutions is 45 mL (adult dose)
    - Two doses of 45 mL can be taken at 24-hour intervals
    - Concomitant use of rehydration solutions increases safety and tolerance by reducing risk of dehydration, electrolytic imbalance, and intravascular volume contraction
    - Onset of action: 30 minutes–1 hour
  o Enema:
    - Bottle of 130 mL solution, fitted with a lubricated rectal cannula (100 mL solution contains 16 g sodium phosphate monobasic and 6 g sodium phosphate dibasic)
    - Recommended use of product in genupectoral position or in a left side-lying position with right knee bent
    - Insert cannula into the rectum, and squeeze the bottle slowly so as to inject the desired quantity
    - Retain solution as long as possible
    - Onset of action: 2–5 minutes
  o Contraindications: renal failure, heart failure, gastro-intestinal occlusion, advanced liver diseases

- o Precautions: elderly persons, patients with reduced gastric motility, low-sodium diet, pre-existing electrolytic imbalance, patients taking diuretics, and/or antihypertensives (ACEIs, ARA), dehydration
- o Side effects: diarrhea, bloating, nausea, hyperphosphatemia, hypokalemia, hyponatremia, decreased serum calcium, acidosis, decreased systolic pressure, spontaneous renal failure with calcification of renal tissues, intestinal erosion
- o Use cautiously with patients having renal failure (risk of hypocalcemia, hyperphosphatemia, hypernatremia, and acidosis) and heart failure (high sodium content: 5 mL = 556 mg Na)

Sodium picosulfate, citric acid, and magnesium oxide (PSMC)

- Reduces absorption of water and electrolytes and increases intestinal motility

- *Pico-Salax*
  - o Two pouches are used. Contents of one pouch are dissolved in 150 mL cold water. Take the first pouch before 8:00 the day before the test, and take the second also the day before the test between 14:00 and 16:00. It is recommended that 250 mL of clear fluids be taken each hour after taking the preparation
  - o Contraindications: heart failure, gastric retention, ileus, gastrointestinal ulceration, gastrointestinal occlusion or perforation, toxic megacolon, severe renal failure, nausea/vomiting
  - o Precautions: elderly or debilitated patients, heart disease, irritable bowel syndrome, patients taking anticonvulsants, patients at risk of electrolytic imbalance caused by medications
  - o Side effects: electrolytic anomalies, dehydration, seizure, hyponatremia, nausea/vomiting, cutaneous rash

References

- Canadian Pharmacists Association. Compendium of Pharmaceuticals and Specialties. 38th edition. Ottawa: Canadian Pharmacists Association; 2003.
- Canadian Pharmacists Association. Compendium of nonprescription products. 7th edition. Ottawa: Canadian Pharmacists Association, 2000.
- Barkun A, Chiba N, Enns R et al. Commonly used preparations for colonoscopy: efficacy, tolerability and safety–A Canadian Association of Gastroenterology position paper. Can J gastroenterol. 2006; 20:699-711.
- Bowles-Jordan J. Constipation. In: Repchinsky C, Leblanc C, editors. Patient self-care: helping patients make therapeutic choices. 1st edition. Ottawa: Canadian Pharmacists Association; Welcom Ltd: 2002. p. 222-37.
- Lum L. Bowel cleansing regimens. Pharmacy practice. 1993; 9:71-7.
- Maher M, Macdonald L. Canadian adverse reaction newsletter. Oral sodium phosphates solutions: electrolyte disturbances. [Internet]. Health Canada. [cited 2006 October 17]. Available from: http://www.hc-sc.gc.ca/dhp-mps/medeff/bulletin/carn-bcei_v12n2_e.html.
- Wexner SD, Beck DE, Baron TH, et al. A consensus document on bowel preparation before colonoscopy: prepared by a task force from The American Society of Colon and Rectal Surgeons (ASCRS), The American Society for Gastrointestinal Endoscopy (ASGE), and the Society of American Gastrointestinal and Endoscopic Surgeons (SAGES). Dis Colon Rectum. 2006; 49:792-809.

Parasites

Head Lice
Pediculosis

Overview

- *Pediculus humanus capitis* parasite infests only humans
- Occurs in 3 forms: nit, nymph, adult louse:
  - Nit: oval, white to yellow, located on hair 1–3 mm above scalp
  - Nymph: tiny louse the size of a pinhead
  - Louse: size of a sesame seed, grey, 6 legs. Usually lives at the back of the head and behind the ears
- Transmission by direct contact and rarely by objects
- Pediculosis commonly occurs in school-age children or pre-schoolers with little relation to personal hygiene or social class
- Close contact (head to head) explains increased incidence of pediculosis in this age group
- Survives 24–48 hours without a host

Questions to ask

- ✓ **What are the symptoms?**
  - Majority of infestations are asymptomatic
  - Itching that usually occurs at the back of the head and behind the ears
  - Differential diagnosis: dandruff, seborrheic keratosis, accumulation of hair product residues
- ✓ **Are there people in the child's family circle who were recently infested?**
- ✓ **How old is the affected child?**
- ✓ **The first episode?**
- ✓ **Any allergies present (chrysanthemum)?**
- ✓ **Other medical conditions (neurological disorder)?**

What to do

- Wash clothes in hot water, then dry them in the drier for at least 20 minutes at high temperature
  - Clothing that can't be washed in hot water can be dry-cleaned or placed in an airtight bag for 10 days
- Vacuum carpets, furniture, and mattresses
- Disinfect personal items (combs, brushes) by soaking them for 5–10 minutes in a bit of undiluted shampoo or in hot water
- Temporarily withdraw child from daycare or school until the pediculosis problem has been resolved
- Avoid use of insecticides available on the market: they are ineffective against pediculosis and can be a health risk for both children and animals
- To remove nits:
  - Apply a moist towel to scalp for 30–60 minutes to facilitate nit removal
  - Divide hair into narrow sections with a fine-toothed comb. Slide the comb from scalp to hair ends
  - It may be necessary to use tweezers or fingernails to remove nits
  - After each comb stroke, soak comb in water to remove lice and nits
  - It is recommended to fine-comb hair every day for a week so as to remove nits during treatment

<u>What to use</u>

- Treat only infested individuals; prophylactic treatment is not advised (increases resistance)

- Repeat treatment in 7–8 days after the first treatment, even if there is no longer a sign of active infestation

- If live lice are visible 24–48 hours after the first treatment, it is recommended that treatment be repeated using a shampoo with a different composition (possible resistance to initial agent)

- Avoid use of conditioners and all-in-one shampoos for a week following treatment so as to avoid reducing residual activity of therapeutic shampoo

- Infected individual remains contagious until all lice and nits have been destroyed

Table I: Pediculicides

	Kwellada-P 1% or Nix 1% (Permethrin) After shampoo	R & C (Pyrethrins and piperonyl butoxide) Shampoo-conditioner	Resultz (Isopropyl myristate and 50% cyclomethicone 5-NF) conditioner	Hexit or PMS-Lindane (Lindane) Shampoo
Classification	Synthetic pyrethroid	Pyrethrin (extract of chrysanthemum insecticide)	Isopropyl myristate	Organochlorine (gamma benzene hexachloride)
Treatment	Pediculosis and pubic lice	Pediculosis and pubic lice	Pediculosis only	Pediculosis and pubic lice
Characteristics	Treatment recommended for children 2 years and older	Synergy with pyrethrins and piperonyl butoxide	Dissolves the wax covering the exoskeleton of lice, causing dehydration and death Indicated for adults and children 4 years and older	Use less and less recommended Not recommended for children under 10 years Second-line treatment
Efficacy	Success rate = 96–100% Powerful insecticide and ovicide Residual effect of about 14 days after treatment	Success rate = 45% after first application; 94% after second application No residual effect so must be repeated in 7–10 days	Success rate = 97% A Phase II study has shown a success rate of 97% by day 21	Success rate = 67–92% Weak ovicide action and no residual effect and so must be repeated after 7–10 days

	Table I: Pediculicides (cont'd)			
	Kwellada-P 1% or Nix 1% (Permethrin) After shampoo	**R & C** (Pyrethrins and piperonyl butoxide) Shampoo-conditioner	**Resultz** (Isopropyl myristate and 50% cyclomethicone 5-NF) conditioner	**Hexit or PMS-Lindane** (Lindane) Shampoo
Precautions	Use cautiously on individuals with chrysanthemum allergies Use by pregnant or breastfeeding women with medical prescription only Avoid contact with eyes and mucosa	Use cautiously on individuals with chrysanthemum allergies Use by pregnant or breastfeeding women with medical prescription only Avoid contact with eyes and mucosa	Eyes must be closed and covered with a towel during application If product comes in contact with eyes, rinse thoroughly with water *Resultz* can create slippery surfaces (floors and bathtubs)	Possible neurotoxicity Contraindicated if history of seizure, large area of excoriated skin, or weight under 50 kg Use of this product with pregnant or breastfeeding women with medical prescription only
Side effects	Itching, erythema, swelling As well, burning sensation, numbness, cutaneous rash	Contact dermatitis caused by petroleum jelly by-products in the preparation	Scalp itching, erythema, and nausea	Benign dermal reactions Neurotoxicity (numbness, nausea, vomiting; seizure)

Table I: Pediculicides (cont'd)

	Kwellada-P 1% or Nix 1% (Permethrin) After shampoo	R & C (Pyrethrins and piperonyl butoxide) Shampoo-conditioner	Resultz (Isopropyl myristate and 50% cyclomethicone 5-NF) conditioner	Hexit or PMS-Lindane (Lindane) Shampoo
Instructions	Wash hair with an ordinary shampoo, rinse with water, and dry thoroughly (do not apply a conditioning product or cream rinse)	Apply sufficient shampoo-conditioner on dry hair to wet it completely	Apply conditioner to dry hair and massage so as to cover from roots to hair ends	Apply sufficient shampoo to dry hair to wet hair completely
	Apply enough after-shampoo to saturate hair and scalp (≈ 25–50 mL)	Leave it on hair for 10 minutes	Leave it on hair for 10 minutes, then rinse with hot water, and wash hair if desired. After that, use a fine comb to remove nits and dead lice	Leave it on hair for 4 minutes
		Add small amount of water until foaming, then rinse thoroughly		Add small amount of water until foaming, then rinse thoroughly
	Leave it on for 10 minutes and then rinse with water		Repeat after 7 days	Repeat after 7–10 days
	Repeat 7–10 days later	Repeat 7–10 days later	Approximate dose by application: Short hair: 30–60 mL Shoulder-length hair: 60–90 mL Long hair: 90–120 mL Do not use on infested eyelashes or eyebrows	For pubic lice, product can be applied for 8–12 hours and then rinsed
				Treatment can be repeated once after 4–7 days

- **Other measures**
  - **Acetic acid, camphor, citronella, sodium lauryl ether sulfate (*SH-206*)**
    - Works both as insecticide and ovicide (according to unpublished studies)
    - Possible development of resistance
    - Benign dermal reactions (3–4%)
    - Not recommended for children under 30 months
    - Repeat after 48 hours and if needed 7–10 days after first application
  - **Permethrin 5% (*Nix*)**
    - Lice resistant to permethrin 1% will also be resistant to stronger concentrations
    - No studies available
    - Apply to dry hair at bedtime. Cover with a shower cap for 10 hours
  - **Combination TMP-SMX and permethrin 1%**
    - Use in cases of repeated failure or for resistant lice
    - By prescription
  - **Occlusive treatment (petroleum jelly)**
    - Suffocates the lice
    - Manual removal of nits essential for treatment to be effective
    - Apply petroleum jelly at bedtime and cover with a shower cap. Repeat every evening for 3–4 days
    - If **eyebrows** are affected, application of petroleum jelly (Vaseline) 3–4 times/day for a week can help to stop infestation
    - Petroleum jelly is difficult to remove once treatment has ended

When to consult

- Persistence of symptoms after 3 treatments in 1 month
- Signs of secondary infection

References

- Buff W. Insect bites and stings and pediculosis. In: American pharmaceutical association handbook of nonprescription drugs. 14th edition. Washington: 2004. p. 889-912.
- Chosidow O. Scabies and pediculosis. Lancet 2000; 355:819-26.
- Flinders DC, De Schweinitz P. Pediculosis and scabies. Am Fam Phys. 2004; 69:341-48,349-50.
- Kaul N, et al. In vivo efficacy and safety of an experimental pediculocide rinse. Hilltop Research Inc, 2004.
- Mansour S. Antiparasitic and anthelmintic products. Carruthers-Czyzewski P, editor. Non-prescription drug reference for health professionals. 1st edition. Ottawa: Canadian Pharmaceutical Association; 1996. p. 101-108.
- Marceau N. Mise à jour sur la pédiculose. Québec Pharmacie. 2004; 51: 773-778.
- Ministère de la Santé et des Services sociaux du Québec. Tout savoir sur les poux de tête. Édition 2002.
- Ministère de la Santé et des Services sociaux du Québec. Protocole d'intervention. July 2000.
- Nycomed Canada. Inc. *Resultz*: Head lice treatment. [Product monograph]. Greensboro. [cited 2006 September]. Available from: http://www.beatheadlice.ca/en/privacy/.
- New over-the-counter head lice treatment: *Resultz*. Pharmacist's Letter/Prescriber's Letter 2006; 22:220919.
- Wendel K, Rompalo A. Scabies and pediculosis pubis: an update of treatment regimens and general review. CID. 2002; 35:S146-51.

Intestinal Worms

Overview

- **Enterobiasis** (*Enterobius vermicularis*, pinworm)

  o <u>Description</u>: This small, round, white worm is 2–5 mm long (male) or 8–13 mm (female) and is responsible for the most common helminth infestation in North America. It especially affects school-age children (age 5–14) without regard to race, culture, or socioeconomic status. About a third of Canadian children will be affected during childhood

  o <u>Transmission</u>: Humans are the only natural host. The parasite is transmitted from one individual to another by egg-contaminated food and air. Eggs can survive up 2 weeks in the environment. When eggs are not reingested, the infestation is self-limiting. A retro-infection (larvae mounting up from the anus) is possible but rare

  o <u>Symptoms</u>: Infestation can be symptomatic or asymptomatic. Nocturnal pruritus (from tickling to acute pain) in the perianal or perineal area can occur when the female deposits its eggs. Infestation can be cyclical, every 2–6 weeks, if there is self-contamination by reingesting eggs. Serious complications are rare (dermatitis, secondary bacterial infection due to scratching, pelvic inflammatory disease, salpingitis, peritonitis, intestinal ulceration, appendicitis)

- **Ascariasis** (*Ascaris lumbricoides* or roundworm)

  o <u>Description</u>: This greyish worm 15–35 cm long is responsible for the most common helminthic infestation in the world. In temperate climates, it mainly affects children and individuals in contact with soil

- o <u>Transmission</u>: Infestation is contracted by ingesting infectious eggs present on fingers contaminated by dirt, food, or dirty water. Eggs remain infectious in the soil for several years. Eggs laid in the intestine are eliminated by bowel movement before they become infectious. Thus, there is no direct transmission between individuals

- o <u>Symptoms</u>: Infection is mainly asymptomatic. Sometimes there are digestive disorders (abdominal pain, nausea, vomiting, diarrhea), some respiratory symptoms (allergic pulmonary reaction, dry cough, expectoration, bronchospasm) or mild fever. Some more serious complications are possible (intestinal occlusion, appendicitis, peritonitis, hepatobiliary ascariasis, pancreatitis)

Questions to ask

- ✓ Who is being treated?
- ✓ Child's age?
- ✓ Pregnant or breastfeeding woman?
- ✓ What are the symptoms? Since when?
- ✓ Worm presence in stool? If yes, collect some and confirm diagnosis with a physician
- ✓ Other individuals living in the same residence?
- ✓ Weight? Allergies? Concomitant medications? (For everyone living in the same place)

What to do

- • Goal: Eradicate the infestation and prevent reinfection
- • Diagnosis must be made before treatment begins

Table I: Diagnostic Methods	
Enterobiasis	Graham Test: In the morning before getting up, firmly apply a 7–10 cm long piece of transparent adhesive tape on the perianal area. Attach the tape, sticky side out, to a glass slide and use a microscope to look for eggs. One sampling detects 50% of infestation, while samplings taken over 3–5 consecutive days detect 90% and 95% of infestations, respectively
	Visual inspection of the perianal area: Using a flashlight, look for a female worm laying eggs, one or two hours after the patient has gone to bed. If possible, collect the worm and place it in alcohol or vinegar and bring it to a physician to confirm the diagnosis
Ascariasis	Under the microscope, examine eggs from stool sample
	Identify an adult worm expelled by bowel movement, vomiting, or spitting. If possible, collect the worm

- If enterobiasis
  - Wash the perianal area each morning in order to eliminate eggs deposited during the night. A shower is preferable to a bath
  - Wash and brush fingernails and hands after going to the toilet and before meals
  - Keep fingernails short
  - Avoid scratching the perianal area. Have children wear appropriate nightclothes to prevent scratching the perianal area
  - Daily washing with hot water (55 °C) of all nightclothes and bedding, particularly after treatment days. Avoid shaking clothes and bedding before washing
  - Daily use of disinfectant for cleaning toilet and bath
  - Daily cleaning of bedroom floors with a vacuum cleaner or moist cloth
  - Keep bedrooms well lit (sunlight kills eggs)
  - Children can return to school after the first treatment dose if fingernails have been cut and cleaned

- If ascariasis suspected
  - Send patient to a physician

What to use

- If enterobiasis
  - Even though infestation may disappear after strict application of hygiene measures, a pharmacological treatment is usually necessary
  - Treat all individuals living in the same residence
  - Repeat treatment of symptomatic persons or those having high risk of reingestion after 2 weeks (agents used do not kill adult worms)
  - Food restrictions and laxative use are not necessary
- If ascariasis
  - First-line treatment is mebendazole (*Vermox*), a prescription drug

Table II: OTC Medications for Treating Enterobiasis and Ascariasis

Medication	Dosage	Adverse Effects	Precautions/Contraindications	Comments
Pyrantel pamoate *Combantrin*	Enterobiasis/Ascariasis 11 mg/kg (base) (maximum: 1 g) X 1 dose Repeat after 2 weeks if enterobiasis 11 mg base = 31.9 mg pamoate	Well tolerated Occasionally: Diarrhea, nausea/vomiting, anorexia Rare: Headache, insomnia, irritability, drowsiness, dizziness, increased AST, ototoxicity, confusion, hallucinations	Pregnancy, breastfeeding, and under 2 years old: few studies so medical opinion necessary Caution if liver failure Avoid if hypersensitivity Interactions: Piperazine (antagonistic effect)	First-line treatment (effective in 90–100% of cases) Can be taken with or without food Little absorption
Piperazine adipate *Entacyl*	Enterobiasis 50–65 mg/kg (hydrate) (maximum: 2.5 g) qd 7 days Repeat 7 days after the end of the first treatment Ascariasis 75 mg/kg (hydrate) (maximum: 3.5 g) qd 2 days 65 mg hydrate = 78 mg adipate	Well tolerated Rare: Gastrointestinal disorders, transient neurotoxicity (paresthesias, drowsiness, lack of coordination, dizziness), hypersensitivity, fever, and joint pain	Pregnancy, breastfeeding, and under age 2: few studies, so medical opinion necessary. Avoid for first treatment but a good choice thereafter, if necessary ** If breastfeeding: discard milk in the 8 hours following each dose** Contraindications: Renal or hepatic dysfunction, seizure disorders, hypersensitivity to piperazine and its salts Interactions: pyrantel (antagonistic effect), phenothiazine (increases risk of extrapyramidal reactions, chlorpromazine (increases potential risk of seizure)	Alternative treatment (effective in 85–90% of cases) Rapidly absorbed and completely eliminated unaltered in urine within 24 hours

When to consult

- All cases where helminthic infection is suspected must be referred to a physician for diagnostic confirmation. This is especially important for:
  - Pregnant or breastfeeding women
  - Children under 2 years or weighing less than 25 kg
  - Patients with renal or hepatic failure, anemia, or severe malnutrition
  - Symptoms suggesting a complication
  - Vague symptoms and negative visual diagnosis
  - Suspected ascariasis
  - Significant or persistent adverse effects of a medication

References

- Abramowicz M, editor. Médicaments antiparasitaires. La Lettre Médicale.1998; 21:93-104.
- Carruthers-Czyzewski P. Pinworms. In: Repchinsky C, Leblanc C, editors. Patient self-care: helping patients make therapeutic choices. 1st edition. Ottawa: Canadian Pharmacists Association; Welcom Ltd: 2002. p. 294-99.
- Goad JA, Neinstein L. Pinworm Infection. In: American Pharmacists Association: handbook of nonprescription drugs. 14th edition. Washington: American Pharmacists Association; 2004. p. 457-67.
- Grencis RK, Cooper ES. Enterobius, Trichuris, Capillaria, and hookworm including Ancylostoma caninum. Gastroenterol Clin North Am. 1996; 25:579-77.
- Groleau M. Le traitement des vers. Québec Pharmacie. 1985; 32: 337-8.
- Groleau MF. Le traitement des vers. Québec Pharmacie. 1995; 42: 60-3.
- Repchinsky C, editor. Compendium of self-care products: the Canadian reference to OTCs. Ottawa: Canadian Pharmacists Association; 2002-3. p.17.

Pubic Lice

Pubic Lice

<u>Overview</u>

- Morphologically, the pubic louse, or *Phthirius pubis*, looks like a tiny crab

- Extremely contagious: usually transmitted by sexual contact. Transmission by indirect contact (clothes, bedding) also possible but less likely

- Especially affects the genitals but the parasite can more or less spread over the whole body in major infestations

<u>Questions to ask</u>

✓ **What are the symptoms?**
  - o Pruritus
  - o Insomnia and irritability
  - o Can be asymptomatic
  - o Differential diagnosis: seborrheic dermatitis, folliculitis, dermatophytosis

✓ **How long have symptoms been present?**

✓ **First episode?**

✓ **Any intimate relations with a partner who has presented similar symptoms?**

✓ **Any allergies present (chrysanthemum)?**

<u>What to do</u>

- See the chapter "Head Lice"

What to use

• See the chapter "Head Lice"

When to consult

• Recommended to consult a physician, because almost a third of individuals with pubic lice also have a sexually transmitted infection

• Persistence of symptoms despite several treatments (3 treatments in a month)

References

• Buff W. Insect bites and stings and pediculosis. In: American pharmaceutical association handbook of nonprescription drugs. 14th edition. Washington: 2004. p. 889-912.
• Chosidow O. Scabies and pediculosis. Lancet 2000; 355:819-26.
• Flinders DC, De Schweinitz P. Pediculosis and scabies. Am Fam Phys. 2004; 69:341-48,349-50.
• Kaul N, et al. In vivo efficacy and safety of an experimental pediculocide rinse. Hilltop Research Inc, 2004.
• Mansour S. Antiparasitic and anthelmintic products. Carruthers-Czyzewski P, editor. Non-prescription drug reference for health professionals. 1st edition. Ottawa: Canadian Pharmaceutical Association; 1996. p. 101-108.
• Marceau N. Mise à jour sur la pédiculose. Québec Pharmacie. 2004; 51: 773-778.
• Ministère de la Santé et des Services sociaux du Québec. Tout savoir sur les poux de tête. Édition 2002.
• Ministère de la Santé et des Services sociaux du Québec. Protocole d'intervention. July 2000.
• Nycomed Canada. Inc. *Resultz*: Head lice treatment. [Product monograph]. Greensboro. [cited 2006 September]. Available from: http://www.beatheadlice.ca/en/privacy/.
• New over-the-counter head lice treatment: *Resultz*. Pharmacist's Letter/Prescriber's Letter 2006; 22:220919.
• Wendel K, Rompalo A. Scabies and pediculosis pubis: an update of treatment regimens and general review. CID. 2002; 35:S146-51.

Scabies

Overview

- Contagious ectoparasitoid disease caused by the acarid mite *Sarcoptes scabiei*. This parasite can survive and reproduce only on human skin

- Without a host, the adult parasite generally survives 2–3 days, while the life of eggs is quite a bit longer, about 10 days

- The female, who causes the infestation, burrows under the skin where she deposits her eggs. A mite lives on average 4–6 weeks

- Scabies is highly contagious and is transmitted in 95% of cases by direct contact (personal and prolonged). Indirect transmission (toiletries, sheets, etc.) is also possible but much less common

Questions to ask

✓ **What are the signs and symptoms?**

  ○ Difficult to diagnose because signs and symptoms of an infestation are quite similar to those of other diseases

    – Generalized pruritus, especially at night (exacerbated by heat)

    – Cutaneous lesions

      - Scabies burrows (linear or sinuous tracks on the epidermis surface)

      - Cutaneous papular lesions that can be highly excoriated and secondarily infected by *S. aureus*

    – Inflamed lesions

      - Especially in folds (elbow, wrist, axilla, knee, etc.)

      - Face and scalp often remain free of scabies in adults, but not in children

    – Differential diagnosis: atopic dermatitis, insect bites, seborrheic keratosis, impetigo

✓ **How long have symptoms been present?**

- o Incubation period is 3–4 weeks for primary infection or several days for reinfestation

✓ **Any contact with a person recently or currently infested by scabies?**

✓ **Any allergies (chrysanthemum)?**

What to do

- If scabies carrier, avoid all personal body contact with other people

- Wash in hot water all clothes, bedding, and towels used the preceding week, then put them in the dryer set on high for 20 minutes

  - o If some clothes cannot be heat dried, put them in a tightly sealed plastic bag for at least 5 days, or dry clean them

- Vacuum furniture and carpets

- If a child is affected, inform child's daycare or school. The child cannot return to school until he or she has been treated

What to use

- A definitive diagnosis must be made by a physician before beginning treatment

- Treatment must be carried out on the infected person as well as on those with whom he or she has been in close personal contact over the last 2 months (symptomatic or not)

- Person infested is no longer contagious 24 hours after treatment. Avoid all contact with others until treatment is completed

- **Permethrin 5%** (*Kwellada-P*, *Nix* **Cream for the skin)**

  - o First-line treatment in adults, pregnant or breastfeeding woman, children, or the elderly

  - o Mechanism of action: inhibits sodium intake in nerve cell canals of the parasite causing its paralysis and death

- Contact time necessary: 8–14 hours
- Single application is appropriate
- Toxicity 40 times less than Lindane
- <u>Side effects</u>: pruritus, erythema, and transient edema
- Avoid use if pyrethrin or chrysanthemum allergies
- Can be used under medical supervision with 2-month-old infants
- If used with children, it should also be applied on the head

- **<u>Lindane 1%</u> (*Hexit, PMS-Lindane*)**
  - Mechanism of action: stimulates the CNS, causing parasite seizures and death
  - Contact time necessary: 8–12 hours
  - A number of clinicians recommend a second application 1–2 weeks after the first to increase treatment efficacy
  - Side effects: local irritation, systemic effects (such as nausea/vomiting, headache, convulsions) if absorbed (liposoluble medication, hence absorption of about 10%)
  - Not recommended for children under 2 years, pregnant women, the elderly, or persons with altered cutaneous barrier
  - Since there is higher resistance to lindane, it is a second-line treatment choice

- **<u>Crotamiton</u> (*Eurax* 10% cream)**
  - Efficacy in only 50–60% of patients with scabies
  - Useful in pediatrics for treating scabies nodules
  - Contact time: 24 hours
  - A second application must be made the next day for another 24 hours of contact time. Take a bath 48 hours after the first application

- **<u>Sulfur</u> (6–10% with petroleum jelly)**
  - Treatment option for pregnant or breastfeeding women and for infants under 2 months
  - Preparation is applied daily for 3 days, 24-hour duration
  - Disagreeable odour and possible local irritation

Table I: Cream Application for Treating Scabies

- Before product is applied, the skin must be clean, dry, and cool
- Spread cream or lotion in quantity sufficient to **cover the whole body surface:** from neck to toes
  - o Remember to carefully apply the product between fingers and toes, on fingernails and toenails, on wrists, axillae, genital and buttocks area, all of which are the most common areas of infestation
- Leave product in place for 12–14 hours (e.g., all night)
- Rinse off product by taking a shower or bath
- Wear clean clothes
- One application is appropriate
  - o Repeat the treatment 7–10 days later only if the parasites are still present or if new lesions appear (unless contraindicated for lindane and crotamiton)
- Pruritus can persist for as long as 4 weeks after the antiparasitic treatment and the elimination of all mites. Their disappearance is usually gradual
  - o Diphenhydramine can help to relieve pruritus
  - o Topical corticosteroids or some cream emollients (*Aveeno*) can also relieve pruritus

When to consult

- When scabies symptoms are more or less specific, it is recommended that the diagnosis be made by a physician
- Recurrence of symptoms after 3 treatments within a month
- Signs of secondary infection
- Immunosuppressed patient or young child
- Severe cases

References

- Chosidow O. Scabies and pediculosis. Lancet. 2000; 355:819-26.
- Karthikeyan K. Treatment of scabies: newer perspectives. Postgrad Med J. 2005; 81:7-11.
- Leonard EA, Sheldon IV. Ectoparasitic infections. Clinics in Family Practice. 2005; 7:97-104.
- Mansour S. Antiparasitic and anthelmintinc products. In: Carruthers-Czyzewski P, editor. Non-prescription drug reference for health professionals. 1st edition. Ottawa: Canadian Pharmaceutical Association:1996. p. 08-12.
- Poirier V. La gale. Québec Pharmacie. 2001; 48:129-34.
- Flinders DC, De Schweinitz P. Pediculosis and scabies. Am Fam Phys. 2004; 69:341-48,349-50.
- Wendel K, Rompalo A. Scabies and pediculosis pubis: an update of treatment regimens and general review. CID. 2002; 35:S146-51.

Insomnia

Insomnia

Questions to ask

✓ **How long has the patient had sleeping difficulties (more or less than 3 weeks)?**

✓ **Problems of frequent waking or difficulty falling asleep?**

  o If waking up:
    - During the night?
    - Very early in the morning?
    - Duration?

  o If problem falling asleep:
    - Time needed to fall asleep?

✓ **Problem history**

  o Sudden beginning:
    - Changes in family life or bedroom changes?
    - Traumatizing experience?
    - Serious illness?
    - Changes in medication?

  o Persistent:
    - Chronic organic illness?
    - Psychological illness (anxiety, depression, psychosis)?

  o Intermittent:
    - Daytime napping? How long?

✓ **Effect on quality of life?**

✓ **Other causes of insomnia**

  o Age (over 65)?
  o Alcohol consumption? Tobacco use?
  o Starting a night shift?
  o Obesity (apnea)?

- o Bed partner (snoring, moving around at night)?
- o Body position, comfortable bed?
- o Recent travel in another time zone?

Table I: Non-Exhaustive List of Medications That Can Cause Insomnia	
Antihypertensives	
· Calcium channel blockers	· β-blockers (propranolol, atenolol, pindolol)
· Clonidine	· Methyldopa
· Diuretics	
Anticholinergics	
Corticosteroids	
CNS Stimulants	
· Caffeine	
· Methylphenidate	
· Nicotine	
Hormone Supplements	
· Oral hormonal contraceptives	
· Thyroid hormones	
· Progesterone (micronized)	
Sympathomimetics	
· Bronchodilators (terbutaline, salbutamol, salmeterol)	
· Theophylline and xanthine derivatives	
· Pseudoephedrine	
Antidepressants	
· Bupropion	
· SNRIs (venlafaxine, duloxetine)	
· SSRIs	
Antineoplastics	
Other	
· Anticonvulsants	· Levodopa
· Street drugs: cocaine, LSD	· Quinidine

Table II: Non-Exhaustive List of Diseases Possibly Causing Insomnia	
Allergies	Incontinence
Nocturnal angina	Heart failure
Sleep apnea	Ischemic heart disease
Arthritis	Chronic obstructive pulmonary disease
Asthma	Degenerative neurological diseases (Parkinson's and Alzheimer's)
Cancer	Various neurological diseases (i.e., peripheral neuropathies)
Chronic pain	Terminal renal diseases
Benign prostatic hyperplasia	Menopause
Hyperthyroidism	Gastroesophageal reflux
Hypothyroidism	Restless legs syndrome
HIV/AIDS	Gastric ulcer

Adapted from Kupper DJ, Reynolds CF. *Management of Insomnia.* N Engl J of Med 1997; 336: 341-6.

What to do

- Identify cause of insomnia
  - Detailed description of sleep over 2 weeks
- Sleep hygiene
  - Sleep enough to feel rested (without sleeping too much)
  - Create an environment favourable to sleeping (eliminate stimuli)
  - Don't take naps during the day. If a catnap is needed, take 30-minute catnap before noon
  - Do relaxation exercises
  - If necessary, have a light snack before bedtime to avoid getting hungry
  - Exercise regularly, but at least 3–4 hours before retiring
  - Avoid caffeinated drinks in the afternoon
  - Avoid alcohol consumption after supper

- o If possible, stop smoking. If not possible to stop, avoid smoking in the evening
- o Do not look at the clock at night
- o Wake up at the same time every morning
- Control of stimuli
  - o Go to bed only when you are ready to sleep
  - o Establish a regular sleep schedule
  - o Reserve bed strictly for sleeping or for sexual activity (avoid watching TV, eating or working in bed)
  - o Leave the bedroom if you are not asleep in 10 minutes. Return to the bedroom when ready to sleep

<u>What to use</u>

- Treatment with medication should be occasional only and for short periods (2–4 weeks)
- Use the smallest effective dose
- Tolerance, dependence, or rebound insomnia can set in with regular use
- Sleep aids do not improve the quality of sleep

Table III: OTC Medications for Treating Insomnia					
Ingredient	**Commercial Names**	**Dosage**	**Onset of Action**	**Side Effects**	**Comments**
Diphenhydramine	*Calmex* *Dormex* *Dormiphen* *Nytol* *Sominex* *Unisom* *Simply Sleep* *Sleep Aid* *Sleep-Eze*	25–50 mg hs	60–180 minutes	Dizziness Change in alertness Anticholinergic effects (dry mouth, constipation, urinary retention)	Tolerance with repeated use Interactions with CYP2D6 Contraindication: closed-angle glaucoma, urinary tract obstruction (including prostatic hyperplasia), hyperthyroidism, asthma, Chronic obstructive lung disease, peptic ulcer with stenosis, pyloroduodenal obstruction Use with caution in patients taking sedatives Side effects can be more pronounced in elderly patients
Doxylamine	*Unisom-2*	25 mg hs	60–120 min	Residual effects possible the following day (due to long half-life)	

Adapted from Kupper DJ, Reynolds CF. Management of Insomnia. N Engl J of Med 1997; 336 (5): 341–6

When to consult

- Insomnia in a child
- Pregnant or breastfeeding women
- Diseases affecting sleep
- Sleep apnea or significant snoring
- Obesity (BMI greater than 35)
- Significant impact on quality of life
- Inefficacy of OTC drug treatment (pharmacological and nonpharmacological) after 14 days
- When a prescription drug or a medical condition seems to be the cause of insomnia
- Contraindications for OTC drugs for treating insomnia

References

- Bureau of Nonprescription Drugs. Sleep aids—labelling standard. [Internet]. Canada. [Updated 1993 July 12, cited 2007 April 10]. Available from: http://www.hc-sc.gc.ca/dhp-mps/alt_formats/hpfb-dgpsa/pdf/prodpharma/slee_somn_e.pdf
- Chokroverty S. Evaluation and treatment of insomnia. [Internet]. UpToDate. [cited 2007 April 4] Available from: http://utdol.com/utd/content/topic.
- Eddy M, Walbroehl GS. Insomnia. Am Fam Physician. 1999; 59 : 1911-6.
- Fleming J. Insomnia. In: Gray J, editor. Therapeutic choices. 3rd edition. Ottawa: Canadian Pharmacists Association; 2000. p. 43-51.
- Kupper DJ, Reynolds CF. Management of insomnia. N Engl J Med.1997; 336:341-6.
- Naidoo S. Sleep aids and stimulants. In: Carruthers-Czyzewski P, editor. Non-prescription drug reference for health professionals. 1st edition. Ottawa: Canadian Pharmaceutical Association; 1996. p. 585-6.
- Ringdahl EN, Pereira SL et Delzell JE. Treatment of primary insomnia. J Am Board Fam Pract. 2004; 17:212-9.
- Sateia MJ, Nowell PD. Insomnia. Lancet. 2004; 364:1959-73.
- Vaillancourt R. Insomnia. In: Repchinsky C, Leblanc C, editors. Patient self-care: helping patients make therapeutic choices. 1st edition. Ottawa: Canadian Pharmacists Association; Welcom Ltd: 2002. p. 49-57.

Ophthalmic Conditions

Blepharitis

Overview

- Chronic or acute inflammation of the eyelid margin
- Possible causes of blepharitis:
  - Bacteria: *Staphylococcus aureus* or *epidermidis*
    - Formation of rings around eyelashes. Produces dry-looking crusts
  - Seborrheic hypersecretion:
    - Oily and yellowish adhesive crusts
  - Irritation or allergy:
    - Ophthalmic medications (atropine, neomycin, pilocarpine, tetracaine, timolol), smoke, dust, cosmetics, plants (ragweed), metal frames of eyeglasses
  - Parasite: pediculosis

Questions to ask

✓ **Presence of symptoms:**
  - Crusts at eyelash base
  - Redness of eyelid margin
  - Sensation of foreign object or burning on eyelid margin
  - Pruritus
  - Tearing
  - Unilateral or bilateral

What to do

- Soften the crusts: apply warm, moist compresses bid–qid 5–15 minutes

- Eyelid hygiene:
  - Prepare a soapy solution (see Table I) or use a commercial product like *Lidcare*

Table I: Preparing a Diluted Soapy Solution	
Ingredient	**Quantity**
Baby shampoo	5 mL (1 tsp.)
Warm water	5 mL (1 tsp.)
Recommended final dilution (shampoo/water): 1:1–1:5	

  - Keep eyes closed
  - Gently rub the eyelid margin with a cotton swab, a washcloth, or gauze soaked with diluted solution
- If necessary, continue hygiene measures above until symptoms disappear, and after as needed
- In case of recurrent inflammation: continue nonpharmacological measures for at least 1 month. Consult an eye care professional
- In case of chronic inflammation: once the acute problem has been resolved, continue hygiene measures daily to prevent recurrence

What to use

- If bacteria suspected:
  - *Polysporin* ointment qid 1–2 weeks (then hs 4–8 weeks in cases of chronic or recurrent blepharitis)
  - Apply after cleaning eyelids (see nonpharmacological measures)
- If seborrheic hypersecretion:
  - Dilute selenium sulfide (*Selsun*) 1:5–1:10 with water, then remove crusts with this solution. Avoid contact with the eye
  - Artificial tears bid–qid can help to reduce debris
- If allergy suspected:
  - Cold compresses + systemic antihistamines

- If pediculosis:
  - Treatment for body lice plus petroleum jelly on lid margins during treatment time

When to consult

- Recurrent or persistent blepharitis
- For all ophthalmic problems, medical consultation necessary as soon as patient presents with one of the following symptoms:
  - Pain
  - Photophobia
  - Altered vision
  - Redness directly around the cornea
  - **Severe** redness of the conjunctiva or eyelids
  - Abnormal pupils (myosis or mydriasis, oval shape, etc.)
  - Trauma
  - Accompanying headaches
  - Black or fuzzy spot in visual field (sudden appearance)
  - OTC products for more than 48–72 hours without improvement

References

- Trottier LR, Wing DS. Eye care products: Disorders of the eyelids. In: Carruthers-Czyzewski P, editor. Non-prescription drug reference for health professionals. 1st edition. Ottawa: Canadian Pharmaceutical Association; 1996. p 167-9.
- Carter SR, Eyelid disorders: diagnosis and management. Am Fam Physician. 1998; 57:2695-702.
- Kaiser PK, Friedman NJ, Pineda R, editors. The Massachusetts eye and ear infirmary illustrated manual of ophthalmology. 2nd edition. Philadelphia: Saunders; 2004.
- Anonymous. Common problems of the eye. [Internet]. Ottawa: Health Canada: Clinical practice guidelines for nurses in primary care; First Nations and Inuit Health. [cited 2007 April 23]. Available from: http://www.hc-sc.gc.ca/fnih-spni/pubs/nursing-infirm/2000_clin-guide/chap_01b_e.html.

Conjunctivitis
Conjunctivitis

Overview

- Inflammation of the eye conjunctiva caused by virus, bacteria, allergies, or irritants

Questions to ask

✓ **How long have the symptoms been present?**

✓ **Symptoms: redness, pruritus, burning sensation or sensation of presence of foreign object, exudate, photophobia (see Table I)**

  ○ If exudate: serous, mucoid, purulent (see Table II)

✓ **Changes in visual field or blurred vision**

✓ **Unilateral or bilateral (often becomes bilateral after 48 hours)**

✓ **Contact lenses?**

✓ **Medication history?**

✓ **Applying medications or topical ophthalmic products?**

✓ **Applying makeup on eyelid or around the eye?**

Table I: Symptoms According to Cause of Conjunctivitis			
Symptoms	**Viral**	**Bacterial**	**Allergic**
Pruritus	Minimal	Minimal	Significant
Redness	Significant	Significant	Significant
Tearing	Significant	Moderate	Moderate
Exudate	Moderate	Abundant, especially in the morning	Moderate
Periauricular adenopathy	Frequent	Rare	Absent
Sore throat and fever	Occasional	Occasional	Absent

Table II: Conjunctivitis and Quality of Ocular Exudate				
Etiology	Serous	Mucoid	Mucopurulent	Purulent
Viral	X			
Chlamydia		X	X	
Bacterial			X	X
Allergic	X	X		
Toxic	X	X	X	

Viral conjunctivitis

What to do

- Reduce risk of transmission: avoid contamination of the area (isolation if necessary) for 7 days starting with first symptoms (highly contagious)
- Wash hands frequently with soap and water before and after any contact with eyes

What to use

- Apply cold water compresses
- Topical ophthalmic antibiotics are not effective

When to consult

- If secondary to herpes simplex or if moderate to severe
- If no improvement after 7–10 days

Bacterial conjunctivitis

What to do

- Bacterial conjunctivitis often resolves spontaneously within 7–10 days
- Clean eyelid with moist gauze or pad

What to use

- Reasons for treating bacterial conjunctivitis: to avoid transmission, reduce infection period, reduce the risk of complications (low risk in a healthy population)
- Topical ophthalmic antibiotics:
  - *Polysporin* drops (polymyxin + gramicidin)
  - *Polysporin* ointment (polymyxin + bacitracin)
- Dosage: apply qid 5–7 days
- Drops will keep 4 weeks after opening; ointment, 3 months

When to consult (see also Table III)

- If presence of pain, photophobia, or blurred vision
- If *Neisseria sp.* or *Chlamydia sp.* suspected (history of STIs, tendency to recur, seropurulent secretion)
- Very young child
- Elderly patient
- If no improvement after 24–48 hours treatment
- Treatment failure (no resolution after 48–72 hours treatment)

Allergic conjunctivitis

What to do

- Identify allergenic agents and avoid exposure to them
- Avoid rubbing eye
- Apply cold water compresses

What to use

- If patient also presents with non-ophthalmic symptoms (rhinorrhea, nasal congestion, etc.): systemic antihistamine (see the section on allergic rhinitis in the chapter "Common Cold, Influenza, and Allergic Rhinitis")
- If patient presents only with ophthalmic symptoms:
  - Artificial tears: lubricate the conjunctiva, produce protective film on the eye, and dilute allergen present on eye so as to reduce contact
    - Dosage: apply 4–6 times/day (see the chapter "Dry Eye")
  - Antihistamines in ophthalmic solution: provide more rapid relief than oral antihistamines
    - Antazoline (*Albalon-A*, *Vasocon-A*)
    - Pyrilamine (*Prefrin-A*)
    - Pheniramine (*Naphcon-A*, *Visine Advance Allergy*, *Opcon-A*)
    - Dosage: apply tid–qid prn
    - Warning: all OTC antihistamines in format of ophthalmic drops are also combined with a decongestant, hence use them no more than 3 days to prevent rebound redness
  - Mast cell stabilizers:
    - Sodium cromoglycate (*Cromolyn*)
    - Onset of action (14 days), slower than ophthalmic antihistamines
    - Dosage: apply qid prn

- o Decongestants in ophthalmic solution:
  - – Reduce redness, but short acting
  - – Naphazoline (e.g., *Clear Eyes*, *Vasocon*)
  - – Oxymetazoline (e.g., *Visine Workplace*, *Claritin Eye Allergy Relief*)
  - – Phenylephrine (e.g., *Mydfrin*, *Prefrin*)
  - – Tetrahydrozoline (e.g., *Visine Original*, *Visine Allergy*)
  - – Dosage: apply tid–qid prn, maximum 3 days, because can produce rebound hyperemia (*conjunctivitis medicamentosa*)
  - – Contraindications: damaged cornea or closed-angle glaucoma
  - – Precautions: if uncontrolled hypertension, diabetes, uncontrolled hyperthyroidism, heart disease, taking tricyclic antidepressants, monoamine oxidase inhibitors, or beta-blockers

When to consult

Table III: Symptoms Requiring Eye Care Professional (overview)	
Intense ocular pain (especially if unilateral)	Abnormal corneal light reflection
Photophobia	Anomaly or opacity of corneal epithelium
Persistent blurred vision	Non-reaction of pupil to direct light
Proptosis (exophthalmia)	Weakened immunity (e.g., newborns, immunosuppressed patients, soft contact lense wearers)
Reduced ocular movement	
Ciliary congestion	

References

- Trottier LR, Wing DS. Eye care products: Disorders of the eyelids. In: Carruthers-Czyzewski P, editor. Non-prescription drug reference for health professionals. 1st edition. Ottawa: Canadian Pharmaceutical Association; 1996. p 170-6.
- Leibowitz HM. The red eye. N Engl J Med. 2000; 343:345-51.
- Morrow GL, Abbott RL. Conjunctivitis. Am Fam Physician.1998; 57: 735-46.
- Anonymous. Assessment of the eyes. [Internet]. Ottawa: Health Canada: Clinical practice guidelines for nurses in primary care; First Nations and Inuit Health. [cited 2007 April 23] Available from: http://www.hc-sc.gc.ca/fnih-spni/pubs/nursing-infirm/2000_clin-guide/chap_01a_e.html.
- Titcomb LC. Over-the-counter ophthalmic preparation. PJ. 2000; 264 (7082):212-18.

Contact Lens Care

Questions to ask

- ✓ Are contact lenses soft or semi-rigid?
- ✓ How often are lenses changed (daily, monthly, annually)?
- ✓ What is the care regimen? Recent changes?
- ✓ Discomfort when putting in the contact lenses (redness, stinging)?
- ✓ Wearing lenses throughout the night?
- ✓ Care of the contact lenses?

What to do

Contact lens care

- Wash hands with soap and water before touching the contact lenses

- Never rinse contact lenses with drinking water or household cleaning products, or personal hygiene products (e.g., toothpaste)

- Rinse the storage case (using a recommended product) and replace the lens solution each time lenses are removed

- Discard all ocular solutions 3 months after opening (for ophthalmic drops, 1 month after opening) even if the product has not expired (so as to ensure the sterility of the product)

- If a care system works well, keep using it unless otherwise advised by an eye care professional

- If change of care system is desired, use new products with new lenses to avoid possible incompatibilities between the different products

- Change contact lens storage cases every 3 months, or clean once a month in the dishwasher, or boil in water for 10 minutes (the *Clear Care* storage case must be replaced every 3 months)

Wearing contact lenses

- Wear contact lenses maximum 10–12 hours/day
- Do not sleep wearing contact lenses
- When swimming, do not wear contact lenses when putting head under water. Wait 1 hour after swimming before putting in lenses
- Notify pharmacist that you are wearing contact lenses; several drugs can interact with contact lenses (Table I)
- Remove contact lenses when applying ophthalmic solutions or ointments to eyes
- Notify an eye care professional when you start taking a new medication

Table I: Interactions Between Medications and Contact Lenses	
Medications	**Description of Interaction**
All topical ophthalmic medications	Can cause: · Eye toxicity · Deterioration of the contact lens · Incompatibility with lens care solution
· Oral contraceptives · Antihistamines · Anticholinergics · Tricyclic antidepressants · Beta blockers · Diuretics	Decrease in tear volume
· Reserpine · Cholinergic agents	Increase in tear volume

Table I: Interactions Between Medications and Contact Lenses	
Medications	**Description of Interaction**
• Phenylephrine, epinephrine (topical), tetrahydrozoline and fluorescein (topical product) • Rifampin • Phenazopyridine • Phenolphthalein • Sulfasalazine • Nicotine • Nitrofurantoin	Discolouration of contact lenses
• Oral contraceptives • Clomiphene • Primidone	Eye edema
• Topical diclofenac • Isotretinoin • Salicylates • Gold salts	Eye irritation or inflammation

What to use

- Care system must include the following steps

  o <u>Cleaning</u>: This step removes debris and lipid deposits on the lens. Place several drops on the lens and rub gently for 20 seconds. Rinse the lens well in order to avoid eye irritation. This step is not needed for daily disposable contact lenses

  o <u>Proteolysis</u>: Protein deposits can become embedded in the lens and result in discomfort as well as bacterial growth. An enzymatic agent hydrolizes and dislodges these deposits (use can be optional depending on life expectancy of the lenses and whether or not there is a tendency for deposits to accumulate: use according to instructions of optometrist or ophthalmologist). Note that it is necessary to clean lenses thoroughly before beginning proteolysis. Enzymatic agents in tablet form can be added to multipurpose solutions

  o <u>Disinfecting</u>: This step eliminates bacteria on lens in order to prevent eye infection. Disinfection can be by the thermal method (heat) or the cold method (solutions). This chapter discusses only the cold method

- Cold disinfecting method:
  - o <u>Hydrogen peroxide</u>
    - – Hydrogen peroxide is an effective disinfectant for soft contact lenses. However these care systems are composed of two steps and may require up to 6 hours in order to complete disinfection
    - – Steps:
      1. Immerse lenses in 3% hydrogen peroxide solution. Oxygen released by peroxide acts as a disinfectant
      2. Neutralize peroxide with solution containing a neutralizing agent such as catalase, sodium pyruvate, sodium thiosulfate, or a platinum disk. The neutralization stage is crucial in order to prevent burning or serious cornea irritation. Possible symptoms lasting several hours include pain, photophobia, and redness
    - – N.B.: Do not use multipurpose commercial peroxide solutions to clean contact lenses. Such products can cause contact lens deterioration
  - o <u>Chemical systems</u>
    - – Lenses must be soaked for at least 4 hours before being placed on eye
    - – <u>Storing</u>: This stage includes preserving, storing, and hydrating contact lenses
    - – <u>Rinsing</u>: This stage removes residues or cleaning products before placing lens in eye
    - – Multipurpose solutions can be used regularly
    - – Isotonic saline solutions, with or without preservatives, are also available. They are used to rinse and store lenses (after disinfection)
    - – <u>Multipurpose solutions</u>: Multipurpose systems are most commonly used because of their practicality. However, their functions (e.g., cleaning and rinsing) are sometimes incompatible. In addition, it is difficult to produce a formulation that contains optimal concentrations of each ingredient without impacting product stability.

Consequently, multipurpose solutions can compromise efficacy of each step of the lens care system. To compensate for this, it is recommended to rub lenses even if using a "non-rub" solution

- Preservatives:
  - o Irritants: thimerosal, chlorhexidine
  - o Agents for sensitive eyes: polyquad, dymed
  - o Several preservatives are incompatible (e.g., chlorhexidine and thimerosal can cause a keratopathy known as "mixed solution syndrome"
- Hard lenses:
  - o Use a system designed for hard lenses. If a change in care regimen is necessary, best is to consult an optometrist or optician

When to consult

- Presence of redness, pain, or sensitivity to light; and in case of loss of vision, or swelling around eye
- If patient is using a hydrogen peroxide care system and presents with the symptoms above, advise patient to remove lenses and rinse eyes with a regular sterile saline solution. If symptoms persist, consult an eye care professional

References

- Trottier LR, Wing DS. Eye care products: Contact lens care. In: Carruthers-Czyzewski P, editor. Non-prescription drug reference for health professionals. 1st edition. Ottawa: Canadian Pharmaceutical Association; 1996. p. 188-198.
- Engle JP. Care of soft contact lenses. [Internet]. US Pharmacist. 2002. [cited 2007 April 4] Available from: http://www.uspharmacist.com/oldformat.asp?url=newlook/files/cons/acf2ff4.cfm.
- Lapierre M, Quesnel NM. Les lentilles cornéennes et solutions. Les agents diagnostiques et thérapeutiques oculaires. Complete edition. Montréal: Université de Montréal; 2003.
- Société canadienne d'opthalmologie. Communiqué de presse. [Internet]. Vaughan,ON. [cited 2007 April 4]. Available from: http://www.eyesite.ca/

Dry Eye

Overview

- Cause of dry eye is often multifactorial. Some common causes are decreased tear production and rapid evaporation of tears

- Working in front of a computer screen can decrease blinking frequency thus decreasing tear production

- Some medications can decrease tear volume:
  - Antihistamines
  - Anticholinergics
  - Tricyclic antidepressants
  - Beta-blockers
  - Diuretics
  - Tretinoin

- Some eye or systemic diseases can be associated with dry eye, for example:
  - Keratoconjunctivitis sicca
  - Chronic conjunctivitis
  - Vitamin A deficiency
  - Hyperthyroidism (with ophthalmopathy)
  - Bell's palsy (facial paralysis)
  - Rosacea
  - Stevens-Johnson syndrome
  - Sjögren's syndrome
  - Eye trauma

Questions to ask

✓ **Symptoms (often exacerbated by wind or smoke)**

- o Dryness or inability to produce tears
- o Overproduction of tears (lacrimation)
- o Redness (moderate to severe)
- o Burning sensation in the eyes
- o Sensation of a foreign object in the eyes
- o Blurred vision
- o Pruritus
- o Difficulty opening and closing eyelids

What to do

- Cold moist compresses for burning sensation
- Humidify rooms
- Lower the room temperature
- Wear protective goggles as needed
- Wear goggles when swimming
- Avoid prolonged wearing of contact lenses (maximum 10–12 hours/day

What to use

Table I: Artificial Tears Available as Eye Drops			
Name	**Preservatives**	**Relative Viscosity**	**Composition**
Cellufresh	-	+	
Refresh	-	+	Polyvinyl alcohol, povidone
Refresh Plus	-	+	Carboxymethylcellulose, sodium lactate
Genteal Mild	-	+	
Moisture Drops	+	+	Hydroxypropyl methylcellulose, povidone, glycerin
Genteal	+	+	
Hypotears	+	+	Polyvinyl alcohol, propylene glycol
Murine	+	+	Polyvinyl alcohol, povidone
Refresh Tears	+	+	Carboxymethylcellulose, sodium lactate
Tears Naturale	+	+	Hydroxypropyl methylcellulose, dextran
Tears Naturale II	+ (Polyquad)	+	Hydroxypropyl methylcellulose dextran
Tears Naturale Free	-	+	Hydroxypropyl methylcellulose, dextran
Isopto Tears 0.5% or 1%	+		Hydroxypropyl methylcellulose 0.5% or 1%
Bion Tears	-	++	Hydroxypropyl methylcellulose, dextran
Refresh Endura	-	++	
Refresh Celluvisc	-	+++	
Murocel	+	+++	Carboxymethylcellulose, propylene glycol
Ultra Tears	+	+++	
Tears Naturale Forte	+ (Polyquad)	+++	Hydroxypropyl methylcellulose, dextran, glycerin

- Eye lubricants
  - Useful for prolonged action
  - Apply at bedtime because of blurred vision after application (e.g., *Duolube* = 90% petroleum jelly)

Table II: Artificial Tears Available as Ointment or Gel	
GenTeal Gel	*Moisture Eyes*
Tears Again	*Refresh PM*
HypoTears	*Tears Naturale PM*
Lacrilube	*Duolube*
Lacrinorm	*Hylashield*

- Life expectancy:
  - Ophthalmic solutions: 4 weeks after opening
  - Nebules: if not opened, to expiry date
  - Ophtalmic ointments: 3 months
  - Eye wash preparations: 1 week after opening

When to consult

- Chronic or persistent symptoms for 72 hours or longer despite treatment
- Presence of chronic or known eye disease

References

- Trottier LR, Wing DS. Eye care products: Dry eye. In: Carruthers-Czyzewski P, editor. Non-prescription drug reference for health professionals. 1st edition. Ottawa: Canadian Pharmaceutical Association; 1996. p. 177-180.
- Kaiser PK, Friedman NJ, Pineda R, editors. The Massachusetts eye and ear infirmary illustrated manual of ophthalmology. 2nd edition. Philadelphia: Saunders;2004.
- Lapierre M, Quesnel NM. Les lentilles cornéennes et solutions. Les agents diagnostiques et thérapeutiques oculaires. Montréal: Université de Montréal; 2003.

Styes

Hordeolum

Overview

- A stye is often caused by *Staphylococcus aureus* infection
- A stye occurs most often on the upper eyelid, near the eyelid margin and eyelashes, but it can also occur on the lower eyelid
- Recurrence rate: 20%
- Not to be confused with a chalazion

Questions to ask

✓ **Symptoms?**

- o Furuncle at eyelash base (eyelash follicle) or in a sebaceous gland (Zeis gland) or apocrine sweat gland (Moll gland)
- o Eyelid inflammation, edema, redness
- o Acute pain at the stye site (chronic stye can be painless)
- o Unilateral or bilateral
- o Single or multiple
- o Often seen as complication of blepharitis

What to do

- Apply hot, moist compresses and massage gently 10–15 minutes tid–qid until symptoms disappear completely
- Do not try to open and drain the stye yourself
- Spontaneous reabsorption in 7–10 days
- Wash hands often to avoid spreading infection

- Avoid cosmetics during acute phase
- Avoid wearing contact lenses during acute phase
- Avoid recontamination: eye makeup used before infection must be discarded

What to use

- ***Polysporin* ophthalmic ointment**
  - To be used only when inflammation extends beyond stye or when stye breaks open and drains
  - Prevents spreading of infection
  - Apply qid after compresses
  - Ointment is preferred because it offers better coverage than an anti-*Staphylococcus aureus* ophthalmic solution

When to consult

- Vision disorders
- Presence of multiple styes
- No improvement after 48 hours of treatment
- Rapid increase in stye size
- Infection spreads in the form of periorbital cellulitis (emergency)
- See the chapter "Blepharitis"

References

- Anonymous. Information générale: Vos yeux et votre vision. [Internet]. Quebec: Association des optométristes du Québec [cited 2007 April 23]. Available from: http://www.aoqnet.qc.ca/public/informations/maladiesYeux.php#7.
- Trottier LR, Wing DS. Eye care products: Disorders of the eyelids. In: Carruthers-Czyzewski P, editor. Non-prescription drug reference for health professionals. 1st edition. Ottawa: Canadian Pharmaceutical Association; 1996. p. 168-9.
- Carter SR. Eyelid disorders: diagnosis and management. Am Fam Physician. 1998; 57:2695-702.
- Kaiser PK, Friedman NJ, Pineda R, editors. The Massachusetts eye and ear infirmary illustrated manual of ophthalmology. 2nd edition. Philadelphia: Saunders; 2004.
- Anonymous. Dermatological Emergencies [Internet]. Ottawa: Health Canada: Clinical practice guidelines for nurses in primary care; First Nations and Inuit Health. [cited 2007 April23]. Available from: http://www.hc-sc.gc.ca/fnih-spni/pubs/nursing-infirm/2000_clin-guide/chap_01a_e.html.

Ear Care

Cerumen Accumulation
Cerumen Accumulation

Overview
- Cerumen elimination is usually natural and spontaneous
- Risk factors for wax accumulation causing blockage
  - Age
  - Excessive hair in ear canal
  - Hearing aid
  - Overproduction of cerumen
  - Narrow external ear canal

Questions to ask
- ✓ **What are the perceived symptoms?**
- ✓ **Gradual reduction in hearing**
- ✓ **Itching**
- ✓ **Sensation of ear fullness or pressure in the ear**
- ✓ **Discomfort, vertigo, tinnitus**
- ✓ **Possible pain**

What to do
- If accumulation is asymptomatic, do not remove wax
- Assure patient that presence of ear cerumen is not a sign of bad hygiene
- Never use cotton swabs (*Q-tips*); risk of exacerbating symptoms and pushing blockage back into ear
- Place several drops of mineral oil, olive oil, or warm water into the ear (let it act for 15 minutes) bid x 3 days, then loosen wax with some drops of warm water in the ear followed by removal with a bulb syringe designed for this purpose (can be done by physician or nurse). Contraindicated if any possibility of damaging tympanic membrane

Table I: Syringing Technique
· Do not syringe if any possibility of damaging tympanic membrane
· Difficult to do yourself; ask a friend to help you
· Fill syringe with warm water
· Hold a basin below the ear/put a towel on your shoulder
· For an adult, pull up back of ear
· For a child, pull ear back and down
· Place syringe into ear opening
· Direct water gently along base of ear canal; the backwash will push wax outwards

- Prophylaxis:
  - Clean outer ear only with a wet washcloth
  - If recurrence, consider prophylactic dose (2 drops of mineral oil once a week)
  - *Earigate*: isotonic solution indicated as preventive. 1–2 drops 2–3 times a week. For a child under 12 years, use the formulation for children. Contraindicated for child under 6 years

What to use

- Little evidence showing that pharmacological measures are more effective than nonpharmacological measures
- If water or mineral oil are not effective, use same procedure with products below:
- <u>Dichlorobenzene/terebenthine oil</u> (*Cerumol*)
  - Caution in case of peanut allergy (contains peanut oil)
  - Not for continuous use (irritation)
- <u>Carbamide peroxide 6.5%</u> (*Murine Ear Drops*)
  - Not for continuous use (irritation)
  - Helps to break down wax by mechanical action

- Triethanolamine polypeptide oleate condensate (*Cerumenex*)
  - Associated with severe hypersensitivity reactions. Perform a patch test before use
  - Follow in 10–15 minutes by syringing
- Hydrogen peroxide 3% diluted 1:1 with warm water
  - Same mechanism as carbamide peroxide
  - Do not use with patients having excessive exfoliation in the ear canal
- Anhydride glycerin
  - Cerumenolytic
  - Use as emulsifier to soften wax. Less effective than carbamide peroxide
  - Safe and non-sensitizing
- Sodium docusate (*Colace*)
  - Solution 10 mg/mL
  - Dosage: 1 mL 10–15 minutes before trying to remove wax
  - Not recommended because more expensive, not very effective, can cause erythema
- Ear candle (not legally available in Canada)
  - Acts by creating negative pressure in external ear canal
  - Do not recommend because it is ineffective and hot wax can damage ear
- All are contraindicated if possibility of damaging tympanic membrane

When to consult

- Pain in ear: can be a sign of infection, damage to hearing apparatus, or of other diseases of the upper respiratory tract (e.g., tumour, buccal ulcer, tonsillitis, sinusitis)
- Presence of vertigo, dizziness, tinnitus, or rash in ear area
- Treatment suggested does not work in 48 hours

- Discharge of pus, blood, or substances other than wax (wax is an oily brownish or yellowish substance)

- Risk of rupturing tympanic membrane, if less than 6 weeks after ear surgery, presence of tympanostomy tube

- Symptoms related to taking ototoxic drugs (can cause symptoms such as some hearing loss):

  o Aminoglycosides (symptoms can begin to appear after stopping the medications)

  o Loop diuretics in heavy doses

  o Antineoplastics (cisplatin, carboplatin, vincristine, vinblastine)

  o Non-steroidal anti-inflammatory drugs

References

- Dinces EA. Cerumen. [Internet]. Up to date. [cited 2007 April 20]. Available from: http://www.utol.com/application/topic.asp?file=genr_med/26969&type=A&selectedTitle=1~5.
- Facts and comparisons. otic conditions. In: Nonprescription drug therapy: guiding patient self-care. 1st edition. St-Louis: Facts and comparisons; 2002. p. 699-763.
- Guest JF, Greener MJ, Robinson AC. Impacted cerumen: composition, production, epidemiology and management. QJM. 2004; 97:477-88.
- Roland PS, Eaton DA, Gross RD, Wall GM, Conroy PJ, Garadi R, et al. Randomized, placebo-controlled evaluation of Cerumenex and Murine earwax removal products. Arch otolaryngol head neck surg. 2004; 130:1175-7.
- Schering. Earigate FAQ – a safe and natural & effective way to remove ear wax. [Internet]. Schering Canada Inc. [cited 2007 April 28]. Available from: http://www.earigate.ca/en/faq/.
- Shevchuk Y. General ear conditions. In: Repchinsky C, Leblanc C, editors. Patient self-care: helping patients make therapeutic choices. 1st edition. Ottawa: Canadian Pharmacists Association; Welcom Ltd: 2002. p. 181-91.
- Whatley VN, Dobbs CL, Paul RI. Randomized clinical trial of docusate, triethanolamine polypeptide, and irrigation in cerumen removal in children. Arch Pediatr Adolesc Med. 2003; 157:1177-80.

Otitis Externa
Swimmer's Ear

Overview

* Acute and diffuse infection of the external ear canal caused by bacteria (especially *Pseudomonas, Staphylococcus, Bacillus* or *Proteus*) or by fungi

* Impact of water: humidity and heat facilitate tissue maceration in the external ear canal. The breakdown of tissue integrity results in pathogen entry, infection, and inflammation. Water retention increases ear pH (normal pH = 4–5), promoting bacterial proliferation. Note that cerumen absorbs water, thus enabling retention

Questions to ask

✓ **Perceived symptoms?**

✓ **Itching or pain in the ear (especially when moving the pinna or jaw)**

✓ **Sensation of liquid in the ear or ear fullness**

✓ **Possible discharge**

✓ **Minor hearing loss possible (linked to inflammation)**

✓ **Fever possible in case of severe infection**

✓ **Itching appears within several hours to 1 day after exposure to water. After that, pain appears and itching increases**

What to do

* Avoid putting head under water when swimming during 7–10 days following a severe infection

* Prevent recurrence if the problem occurs frequently:

  ○ Avoid putting head under water when swimming

  ○ After shower or swim, gently dry ears with a slightly damp washcloth or with a hair dryer at low heat and power

- o Avoid using cotton swabs (*Q-tips*) or any other solid object to clean ears
- o Avoid using earplugs
- o Avoid excessive drying of ears; cerumen protects the ear canal. Remove cerumen from exterior ear canal with a washcloth and warm water and mild soap
- o Use of pharmacological products can act as a preventive measure (see below)

What to use

- Acetic acid 2% (*Vosol*)
  - o Treatment: 4–6 drops qid ad 3 days after symptom disappearance (5–7 days in most cases). Relieves pain and reduces inflammation. Anti-bacterial and anti-fungal activity, acidifying the area. An astringent and a cerumenolytic
  - o Prophylaxis: 4–6 drops after a swim or shower
  - o Keep head bent for 3–4 minutes after application
  - o Do not rinse out drops
- Aluminum acetate 0.5% (*Buro-Sol* otic solution)
  - o Same dosage as acetic acid
- Polymyxin + gramicidin (*Polysporin* otic and ophthalmic solution)
  - o Rapid resistance of *Pseudomonas* (main causal agent)
  - o Treatment: 2 drops in affected ear tid–qid ad 3 days after symptom disappearance (usually 5–7 days)
  - o Do not use as prophylactic
- Home remedy
  - o Prepare a mixture of white vinegar (1:1) with isopropyl alcohol or with propylene glycol
  - o Same dosage as for commercial preparations based on acetic acid or on aluminum acetate
- Analgesics like acetaminophen or ibuprofen can be used to relieve pain (see the chapter "Pain")

When to consult

- Spontaneous loss of hearing

- Bloody or purulent discharges

- Severe pain (especially sudden pain onset linked with discharge, stabbing pain, intolerable pain)

- Tinnitus

- Vertigo

- Swelling and redness spreading outside of the external ear canal

- No improvement after 48 hours of treatment

- Diabetic or immunosuppressed patient (more risk of complications)

- Ear trauma

- Systemic symptoms

References

- Clark WB, Brook I, Bianki D, Thompson DH. Microbiology of otitis externa. Otolaryngol head neck surg.1997; 116:23-5.
- Goguen LA. Otitis externa. [Online]. UpToDate Online. [cited 2007 April 29]. Available from: http://utdol.com/utd/content/topic.do?topicKey=pc_id/2947&type=A&sele ctedTitle=1~9.
- Rosenfeld RM, Singer M, Wasserman JM, Stinnet SS. Systematic review of topical antimiocrobial therapy for acute otitis externa. Otolaryngol Head Neck Surg. 2006; 134:S24-48.
- Rosenfeld RM, Brown L, Cannon CR, Dolor RJ, Ganiats TG, Hannley M et al. Clinical practice guideline: acute otitis externa. Otolaryngol Head Neck Surg. 2006; 134:S4-23.
- Shevchuk Y. Otits externa. In: Repchinsky C, Leblanc C, editors. Patient self-care: helping patients make therapeutic choices. 1st edition. Ottawa: Canadian Pharmacists Association; Welcom Ltd: 2002. p. 192-7.
- Torsher L. Ear Care Products. n: Carruthers-Czyzewski P, editor. Non-prescription drug reference for health professionals. 1st edition. Ottawa: Canadian Pharmaceutical Association; 1996. p. 149-161.
- Van Balen FAM, Smit WM, Zuithoff NPA, Verheij TJM. Clinical efficacy of three common treatments in acute otitis externa in primary care: randomised controlled clinical trial. BMJ. 2003; 327: 1201-5.

Smoking Cessation

Questions to ask

✓ **For whom?**

✓ **What are the real motivations?**

　　○ Is the patient ready to stop smoking?

　　○ How does patient feel when thinking about stopping?

✓ **What are the patient's habits?**

　　○ When, how, or why is the patient smoking? (socially, at work, etc.)

　　○ Number of cigarettes/day?

　　○ How soon after getting up does the patient smoke a first cigarette?

✓ **Has the patient already tried to stop smoking? If yes, what happened? What has the patient tried?**

✓ **Regular medications? If yes, which ones?**

✓ **Chronic health problems?**

✓ **Patient's weight? Less than 45 kg?**

✓ **Calculate nicotine tolerance using the Fagerström Scale if *Nicorette* gum is being considered**

Table I: The Fagerström Nicotine Tolerance Scale				
	A=0 points	B=1 point	C=2 points	Score
How long after you wake up do you smoke your first cigarette?	After 30 minutes	Within 30 minutes		
How many cigarettes a day do you smoke?	1–15	16–25	More than 26	
Does the brand you smoke have a low, medium, or high nicotine content?	Low, less than 0.4 mg	Medium, between 0.5 and 0.8 mg	High, greater than 0.9 mg	
Which of all the cigarettes you smoke a day is the most satisfying one?	Any, other than the first one in the morning	The first one in the morning		
Do you smoke more during the first hours of awakening than during the rest of the day?	No	Yes		
Do you smoke when you are so ill that you are in bed most of the day?	No	Yes		
Do you find it difficult to refrain from smoking in places where it is forbidden, such as the library, theatre, doctor's office?	No	Yes		
How often do you inhale smoke from your cigarette?	Never	Sometimes	Always	

Source: *Nicorette* Gum Product Monograph. Compendium of Pharmaceuticals and Specialties—Canadian Pharmacists Association, 2007.

Table II: Health Benefits of Quitting Smoking: Strategies	
20 minutes after quitting	• Your blood pressure drops to your pre-cigarette level
8 hours after quitting	• The carbon monoxide in your blood drops to normal and the oxygen level in your blood increases to normal
24 hours after quitting	• You lower your chances of having a heart attack
48 hours after quitting	• Your sense of smell and taste improve and begin to return to normal
2 weeks–3 months after quitting	• Your circulation improves and your lungs work better
9 months after quitting	• You experience less coughing, sinus congestion, fatigue, and shortness of breath
1 year after quitting	• Your risk of heart disease is about half of what it would have been if you had continued to smoke
5 years after quitting	• Your risk of stroke is greatly reduced. Within 5–15 years after quitting, it becomes about the same as a non-smoker's risk
10 years after quitting	• Your risk of dying from lung cancer is about half of what it would have been if you had continued to smoke. Your risk of cancer of the mouth, throat, esophagus, bladder, kidney, and pancreas also decreases
15 years after quitting	• Your risk of heart disease is the same as a person who never smoked

Source: Health Canada, Smoking Cessation in the Workplace—A Guide to Helping Your Employees Quit Smoking

http://www.hc-sc.gc.ca/hl-vs/pubs/tobac-tabac/cessation-renoncement/section-6_e.html - 6.1

What to do

- Acupuncture and laser treatment: help to relieve withdrawal symptoms and decrease urge to smoke

- Support groups

- Pre-patch: filter reducing nicotine absorption. No significant clinical efficacy, but increases confidence of some patients

- Strategies dealing with some concerns related to smoking cessation

Table III: Nonpharmacological Measures	
Concerns	**Strategies**
Withdrawal symptoms	· Consider nicotine replacement therapy
Stress management	· Avoid or change sources of stress · Try some relaxation techniques · Take a bath or shower · Go for a walk
Strong urge to smoke	· Seek distraction · Wait 5 minutes before deciding to light a cigarette (these urges usually do not last more than a few minutes) · Drink water or eat raw vegetables · Breathe deeply
Weight gain	· Focus especially on benefits · If appetite increases, drink water and hypocaloric juices, add hypocaloric snacks
Social relations	· Tell friends who are smokers about your decision · Ask for support from family and social network · Go to places where smoking is prohibited

Adapted from: Health Canada, On the road to quitting–Guide to becoming a non-smoker, 2007
http://www.hc-sc.gc.ca/hl-vs/pubs/tobac-tabac/orq-svr/index_e.html

What to use

(See table on nicotine replacement therapies)

- For smoking cessation, there is little evidence that any one nicotine formulation is more effective than another

- Use of a nicotine replacement therapy (NRT) doubles the chance of success

- Recommend not smoking to avoid risks of overdose and to maximize chance of success. If total abstinence is not observed in the first 4 weeks, patch use must be stopped

- Inform patient of withdrawal symptoms. These symptoms appear several hours after smoking cessation, peaking in 48 hours and then gradually decreasing in the following 2–5 weeks

- The polycyclic hydrocarbons in nicotine are inducers of cytochrome P450 isoenzymes. They are inducers mainly of 1A2, 2E1, and 2D6 isoenzymes. It is thus necessary to watch for the effect of smoking cessation on some medications such as theophylline, caffeine, clozapine, olanzapine, insulin, chlorpromazine, warfarin, and beta blockers. A clinically significant effect can be expected in individuals smoking more than 20 cigarettes a day

- Contraindications for all nicotine replacement therapies:
  - o **Recent** history of cardiovascular disease
  - o Arrhythmia
  - o Unstable angina, myocardial infarction
  - o Pregnant or breastfeeding (relative contraindication)

Table IV: Withdrawal Symptoms
Irritability, impatience, nervousness
Difficulty concentrating
Uncontrollable urge to smoke
Headaches
Sleep disturbance
Increased appetite
Tremors, dizziness, increase in appetite

Table V: Nicotine Replacement Therapies (NRTs)

NRT	Dosage	Side Effects	Instructions
Nicotine Gum *Nicorette* *Nicorette Plus* *Thrive gum*	**Points on the Fagerström Scale ≥ 7** **4 mg:** • 1 piece for every 2 cigarettes smoked, ad 20 pieces/day **Points on the Fagerström Scale ≤ 6** **2 mg** • 1 piece per cigarette smoked, ad 20 pieces/day • Also, the amount of gum to use is decided according to the number of cigarettes/day, more or less 20 cigarettes/day, or whether or not the first cigarette is smoked < 30 minutes after getting up • Maximum duration of treatment is 3 months for the initial dose and then gradual reduction of the daily number of pieces over 1–3 months, then use prn	• Mouth and throat irritation • Nausea • Hiccupping • Headache • Indigestion • Dyspepsia • Hypersalivation	• Method: chew, chew, stop for 1 minute • During pause, place the gum between cheek and gums; change placement each time to limit mouth irritation • Discard gum after about 30 minutes of use • Maximum: 20 pieces/day • Do not drink acidic beverages (carbonated drinks, coffee, orange juice) 15 minutes before or during gum use because it alters nicotine absorption

Table V: Nicotine Replacement Therapies (NRTs) (cont'd)

NRT	Dosage	Side Effects
Nicotine Lozenges *Thrive* 1 and 2 mg	**≥ 20 cigarettes/day** · Use the 2 mg lozenges **≤ 20 cigarettes/day** · Use the 1 mg lozenges · In general, 10 lozenges/day are required	· Put lozenge in the mouth and suck lightly unitil it has a strong taste · Then, keep the lozenge between cheek and gums · Wait 1 minute or until the taste disappears, and then repeat sucking until the strong taste returns · Usually a lozenge will melt completely in about 30 minutes. Repeat with another lozenge as needed when an urge to smoke · Lozenges can be used for at least 3 months, as guided by the following table (usage schedule) · After 3 months, the patient must gradually reduce the number of lozenges used each day until he/she stops using the product. Treatment must be terminated when the patient is using no more than 1–2 lozenges/day

Number of cigarettes smoked per day	Weeks 1–2	Weeks 3–4	Month 2	Month 3	Months 4–6
			Lozenges/day		
≥ 20	15	12	10	5	Take 1 as needed if urge to smoke returns
15–19	10	8	5	3	
11–14	7	5	3	2	
≤ 10	5	3	3	2	

Table V: Nicotine Replacement Therapies (NRTs) (cont'd)

NRT	Dosage	Instructions				
		• Put lozenge in the mouth • Let the lozenge melt slowly in the mouth. A sensation of heat or tingling can occur. Do not chew or swallow the lozenge • From time to time, move lozenge from one side of the mouth to the other until lozenge is completely dissolved (20–30 minutes)				
Nicotine Lozenges *Nicorette* lozenges 2 and 4 mg	**If first cigarette of the day is smoked more than 30 minutes after waking:** • Use the 2 mg lozenges **If first cigarette of the day is smoked within 30 minutes of waking:** • Use the 4 mg lozenges	Months 1–3			Months 4–6	
		Weeks1–6	Weeks 7–9	Weeks 10–12	Weeks 13–24	
		1 lozenge/ 1–2 hours Minimum 8 lozenges/day are recommended	1 lozenge/ 2–4 hours	1 lozenge/ 4–8 hours	1–2 lozenges/day if urge to smoke returns	
		Maximum 5 lozenges/6 hours. Do not use more than 15 lozenges/day				

• Overview of nicotine lozenges:

  o Concomitant consumption of acidic beverages such as coffee, tea, carbonated or alcoholic beverages and citrus fruit juices can reduce buccal absorption of nicotine. Avoid drinking acidic beverages 15 minutes before taking a lozenge

  o Side effects are similar to those induced by nicotine absorbed by smoking. At the beginning of treatment, nicotine released by the lozenge can sometimes cause mild throat irritation and an increase in salivation. Initially, excessive ingestion of saliva-released nicotine can cause hiccupping. Individuals subject to indigestion may at the beginning of treatment suffer dyspepsia or minor stomach burning. Usually these effects can be avoided by sucking the lozenge more slowly

Table V: Nicotine Replacement Therapies (NRTs) (cont'd)

NRT	Dosage	Side Effects	Instructions
Inhaler *Nicorette* Inhaler	6–12 cartridges/day up to 12 weeks, then reduce by half for 6–12 weeks, then stop • Maximum duration of treatment: 6 months One 10 mg cartridge represents inhalation period of 20 minutes When cartridge is empty, it usually loses its mint taste	• Cough • Mouth and throat irritation • Aphthous ulcers • Nausea/ vomiting • Hiccups • Headache • Patient must completely stop smoking during the treatment • Side effects decrease with use	• More expensive than other NRTs • Remove the mouthpiece from its envelope • Separate the 2 parts of the mouthpiece, aligning the 2 indicators • Take the cartridge and press it firmly into the lower part of the mouthpiece so as to break open the seal • Line up the top and bottom indicators and press firmly • An opened inhaler cartridge must be used within 12 hours • Do not drink acidic beverages (carbonated drinks, coffee, orange juice) for 15 minutes before and during use to avoid altering nicotine absorption • After using, inhaler cartridge is removed from the mouthpiece and discarded out of children's reach. Store mouthpiece in its box for further use

Table V: Nicotine Replacement Therapies (NRTs) (cont'd)

NRT	Dosage	Side Effects	Instructions
Patches	**>10 cigarettes/day** Begin with 21 mg/day or 15 mg/16 hours	• Headache • Unusual dreams • Insomnia • Patch can be removed at bedtime if the patient has insomnia problems	• Apply on clean, dry skin free of hair (arm, trunk, thigh) • Change application site every day, and wait 1 week before placing a patch in the same place
Nicoderm *Habitrol* Dosage/Patch: 21 mg/24h 14 mg/24h 7 mg/24h	**<10 cigarettes/day or patient weight < 45 kg** Begin with a patch 14 mg/day or 19 mg/16 hour	• Contraindication: cutaneous hypersensitivity to the patch or generalized cutaneous disease	• If redness persists, remove patch after 16 hours or remove at bedtime • Remove patches before any intense physical exercise to avoid intoxication due to increased absorption of nicotine. Increase in skin temperature, vasodilatation, and increased cutaneous blood flow as a result of exercise can have this kind of effect
Nicotrol Dosage/patch 15 mg/16h 10 mg/16h 5 mg/16h	• Treatment period: each stage lasts 2–3 weeks. Decrease gradually over at least 8 weeks of treatment *Note: Nicoderm* and *Habitrol* are not considered equivalent: *Nicoderm* uses a matrix reservoir with a rate-limiting membrane while *Habitrol* uses a gel matrix reservoir. Therefore, only the *Habitrol* patch can be cut if needed.	• If there is redness at the site, rotate sites and apply HC 0.5% cream or use anti-H₁ po	• Patients presenting severe morning withdrawal symptoms are more successful if they wear the patches for 24 hours

When to consult

- If patient presents contraindications to NRTs (note the relative nature of these contraindications because NRTs deliver less nicotine and are less harmful than inhaling smoke):
  - Recent myocardial infarction (within 4 weeks)
  - Unstable or severe angina
  - Severe arrhythmia
  - Recent cerebrovascular accident
  - Allergy to patches or generalized cutaneous disease making it difficult or impossible to use patches
  - Pregnant or breastfeeding (no data on safety)
- Need for non-nicotine treatment (bupropion, varenicline, clonidine, nortriptyline)

References

- Anonymous. *Thrive* Lozenge Product information. [Internet]. Novartis Canada Inc. Mississauga. 2007. Available from: http://thrive.stopsmokingcentre.net/english-site/index.html.
- Anonymous. Product monograph: *Nicorette* lozenge. McNeil consumer healthcare 2007.
- Choquette J., L'abandon du tabac. Québec pharmacie. 2002; 49: 113-23.
- Joseph AM, Norman SM, Ferry LH et al. The safety of transdermal nicotine as aid to smoking cessation in patient with cardiac disease. N Eng J Med. 1996; 335:1792-8.
- Canadian Pharmacists Association. Product monograph: *Nicoderm*. In: Compendium of nonprescription products. 38th edition. Ottawa: Canadian Pharmacists Association. 2007.
- Canadian Pharmacists Association. Product monograph *Nicorette* Inhaler. In: Compendium of nonprescription products. 38th edition. Ottawa: Canadian Pharmacists Association. 2007.
- Product monograph *Habitrol*. [Internet]. Transdermal therapeutic system smoking cessation aid. Novartis Consumer Health Canada Inc. [cited 2007 August 27]. Available from: http://www.habitrol.com.
- Rantucci M., Smoke cessation products. In: Carruthers-Czyzewski P, editor. Non-prescription drug reference for health professionals. 1st edition. Ottawa: Canadian Pharmaceutical Association; 1996. p. 261-74.

- Régie régionale de la santé et des services sociaux. Direction de la santé publique en collaboration avec le Collège des médecins. Lignes directrices: La prévention et l'abandon du tabagisme. January 1999.
- Anonymous. Prenatal and Postpartum Women and Tobacco. [Internet]. Canada: Health Canada. [cited 2007 August 27]. Available from: http://www.hc-sc.gc.ca/hl-vs/pubs/tobac-tabac/prenatale/index_e.html.
- Anonymous. Smoking Cessation in the Workplace—A Guide to Helping Your Employees Quit Smoking. [Internet]. Canada: Health Canada. [cited 2007 August 27]. Available from: http://www.hc-sc.gc.ca/hl-vs/pubs/tobac-tabac/cessation-renoncement/section-6_e.html.
- Zevin S, Benowithz NL. Drug interaction with tobacco smoking. Clin Pharmacokinet. 1999; 36:425-38.

Common Cold, Influenza,
and Allergic Rhinitis

Overview

Cold

- Acute viral infection of the upper respiratory tract

- Synonyms: catarrh, coryza, infectious rhinitis

- Epidemiology: highly contagious, transmission by infectious respiratory secretions, especially "hand-to-hand" contagion, peaking in the fall, mid-winter, and early spring

Influenza

- Acute viral pulmonary infection caused by types A and B *Influenza* virus

- Synonym: flu

- Epidemiology: contagion by infectious respiratory secretions, transmission mainly "hand-to-hand," peaking in winter

Allergic Rhinitis

- Inflammatory disease of the nasal mucous membranes after an antigen-antibody reaction

Table I: Main Conditions of the Upper Respiratory Tract

	Cold	Influenza	Acute Sinusitis	Pharyngitis	Allergic Rhinitis
Etiology	Rhinovirus 30–50% with >100 serotypes Coronavirus 10–15% Less commonly adenovirus, parainfluenza, enterovirus, respiratory syncytial virus	Influenza A (more common; clinical manifestations more severe; serotypes according to 2 antigens: hemagglutinin HA and neuraminidase NA) Influenza B	Viral (rhinovirus; clinical improvement after 7–10 days, clear secretions) Bacterial (*H. influenzae, S. pneumoniae* especially; clinical deterioration after 5–7 days and/or persistence >10 days)	Viral (rhinovirus in 20% cases of common cold evolution; coronavirus 5%; adenovirus 5%; Epstein-Barr; HIV) Bacterial (*Strep. β-hemol.* Group A 15–30% of pharyngitis cases; *Strep. β-hemol.* Group C 5%)	Tree pollen/buds (especially in spring). Grass pollen (end of spring until summer) Ragweed pollen (end of summer until fall) Exterior and/or interior moulds Mites Pets
Transmission /Contagion	Inoculation of nasal mucosa or conjunctiva by hands, contaminated objects and/or through exposure to aerosolized agents; presence of virus in the nasopharynx up to 16–18 days	Inhaling contaminated secretions and/or by various objects (virus survives ad 48h outside of host); contagious after 24–48h ad 5–7 days after beginning of the infection; contagious period longer in children	Secondary infection by flora in most cases	Highly contagious; contagion during and ad 1 week after resolution	Contact of nasal mucosa with an airborne allergen

209

Table I: Main Conditions of the Upper Respiratory Tract (cont'd)

	Cold	Influenza	Acute Sinusitis	Pharyngitis	Allergic Rhinitis
Risk factors	Tobacco use Malnutrition High-density population Sedentariness Chronic psychological stress (> 1 month)	Age extremes Susceptibility of host (genetic factors, innate reactivity of immune system) Virulence of infecting strain	Allergic rhinitis Anatomical abnormalities Recent tooth extraction Recent viral infection of respiratory tract Immuno-suppression	Mostly in children (S. pyogenes or Group A Strep. β-hemol.)	Asthma Atopic diseases Genetic predisposition
Duration	~ 7 days (~25% of cases ad 14 days)	~ 10 days	Variable, several days to several weeks (> 3 months = chronic)	~ 8–10 days if bacterial; shorter duration if viral	Variable depending on allergen involved
Nasal dripping	Present in 45–75% of cases; clear then mucopurulent	Occasionally; clear secretions then mucopurulent	Persistent, purulent coloured rhinorrhea (especially if bacterial)	Present if viral	Frequent; aqueous and clear
Nasal congestion	Present in 45–75% of cases; peaks day 2–3	Occasionally	Persistent	Present if viral	Frequent
Fever	Rare; low fever if present	Appears suddenly, usually lasts 2–3 days; high fever (39–40°C)	Occasionally	Yes, high fever (> 38.8°C)	No

Table I: Main Conditions of the Upper Respiratory Tract (cont'd)					
	Cold	Influenza	Acute Sinusitis	Pharyngitis	Allergic Rhinitis
Sore throat	First symptom; present in 33–50% of cases	Occasionally	Rare	Severe and sudden; accompanied by pharyngeal exudate	Occasionally via pharyngeal inflammation
Cough	Present in < 20% of cases; appears day 4–5, especially a dry cough	Frequent; dry. Appears in first 2 days	Rare	Rare	Occasionally Often involves a post-nasal drip
Headache	Rare	Frequent and severe	Frequent and severe	Rare	Depending on severity; via sinus congestion
Pain/general malaise	Rare; usually minor	Frequent, high intensity and can last ad 2–3 weeks	Pain localized in face and jaw	Possible pain in the inner ear; malaise depending on severity	Pain in the inner ear and in the sinuses; fatigue and malaise depending on severity

	Cold	Influenza	Acute Sinusitis	Pharyngitis	Allergic Rhinitis
Table I: Main Conditions of the Upper Respiratory Tract (cont'd)					
Other features	Typical sequence of symptom appearance (sore throat and malaise/nasal symptoms and cough	Positive predictive value is 85% if presence of cough and fever 36–48h after beginning of infection (useful in determining the target population that could benefit from viral neuraminidase inhibitors; reducing severity and duration of symptoms by ~ 1–1.5 days)		Symptoms suggesting a Group A β-hemolytic *Streptococcus* infection: high fever, sudden, severe sore throat, purulent exudate, swollen/sensitive lymph nodes; diagnosis by special throat culture (sensitivity of the culture > sensitivity of rapid antigen detection)	
Complications	Especially secondary bacterial infection (sinusitis in 0.5–2% of cases of colds, pneumonia, otitis media	Especially secondary bacterial infection (sinusitis, pneumonia, otitis media), viral pneumonia, Reye's syndrome (pediatrics and ASA) rhabdomyolysis (rare, especially in pediatrics)	Affects CNS (meningitis, cerebral abscess), local extension (osteitis of the sinus bone, orbital cellulitis, intracranial infection)	Rheumatic fever (an antibiotherapy begun < 10 days after onset of the infection enables prevention), glomerulonephritis with acute renal failure, local extension (retropharyngeal abscess, otitis media, sinusitis, mastoiditis)	Otitis media, recurrent sinusitis, asthmatic exacerbations, Eustachian tube dysfunction, middle-ear congestion with reduced hearing, chronic sinus pain

Questions to ask

✓ **Description of symptoms**

   o Severity, sequence of appearance, duration, season

   o Symptom variation during the day

   o Secretion and expectorate colour

   o Absence or presence of pus in back of throat

   o Productive or non-productive cough

   o If patient presents only a cough, evaluate:
   - Angiotensin-converting enzyme inhibitors (ACEIs) (incidence 5–35%; can occur with the first dose, but also after several months of use; the effect is not related to the dose; dry cough associated with a prickling, tingling sensation in the throat area)
   - Severe cough, duration < 3 weeks, most usually following pneumonia, a viral infection of the upper respiratory tract, an exacerbation of asthma/COPD, post-nasal drip syndrome, exposure to allergens/irritants, acute bronchitis associated with a productive cough, or more rarely a severe *Chlamydia* or *B. pertussis* infection, a pulmonary embolism, an exacerbation of congestive heart failure.
   - Sub-acute cough, duration 3–8 weeks; in most cases, a post-infectious manifestation (post-nasal drip syndrome, irritation of upper respiratory tract, mucus accumulation due to hypersecretion and/or reduced clearance or bronchial hyperactivity), asthmatic exacerbation, pneumonia, exposure to allergens/irritants
   - Chronic cough, duration > 8 weeks, often multifactorial (gastroesophageal reflux, post-nasal drip syndrome, tobacco use, ACEIs, asthma, nonasthmatic eosinophilic bronchitis, HIV, tuberculosis, a tumour invading an respiratory tract)

✓ **Has the patient any special health problems?**

✓ **Is the patient pregnant?**

<u>What to do</u>

- Bed rest (except for allergic rhinitis)

- Wash hands regularly

- Avoid contaminating surfaces and objects with high risk of transmission

- Drink a lot of water because fever increases unnoticed dehydration (hot and cold fluids). Drink hot beverages such as chicken broth, tea, or hot milk, helping to mobilize nasal secretions

- Increase humidity level in the home (> 50%)

- Use drops (young children) or nasal spray with saline solution NaCl 0.9%. Use a commercial saline solution or a home solution (mix 5 mL table salt with 250 mL warm water) to hydrate the nasal mucosa and to help release viscous secretions

- Gargle with saline solution x 15 seconds q1h (if presence of sore throat)

  o ¼ tsp. salt in 250 mL warm/hot water

- Use petroleum jelly or isotonic-saline-solution based gels to protect irritated perinasal areas

- In case of allergic rhinitis: avoid exposure to allergens

- Pharmacist must promote and encourage vaccination for individuals presenting high risk of influenza-related complications:

  o Adults or children with severe cardiovascular or chronic respiratory diseases requiring regular medical follow-up

  o Any resident of a long-term care facility or other care and housing facilities, regardless of age

  o All persons > 65 years, adults and children with chronic diseases such as diabetes or other metabolic disorders, cancer, immunodeficiency, renal disease, anemia, or hemoglobinopathy

- Pharmacist must encourage judicious use of antibiotics, educating the population as well as early identification of patients who would benefit from antibiotherapy for treating a secondary infection or any other bacterial infection of the respiratory tract

- For pediatric information, consult the chapter "Common Cold and Flu"

What to use

- Most infections of the upper respiratory tract are viral in origin, and thus their treatment is symptomatic

Sore throat

- <u>Lozenges</u>: non-medicated/with anesthetic/with antibiotics/others
  - o salivation (prevents irritation caused by open mouth breathing)
  - o moderate effect
  - o short acting (less than 2 minutes)
  - o Caution: some lozenges contain decongestants and/or cough medication (do not exceed maximum dose)

- <u>Analgesics</u>: ASA/acetaminophen/ibuprofen

Decongestants

- Nasal congestion is caused by a local inflammatory reaction that increases production and secretion of mucus and blood flow as well as vascular permeability (directly by a bacteria/virus or indirectly by histamine release in the case of allergic rhinitis)

- Decongestants have an agonist effect on α_1 receptors of blood vessels, which causes vasoconstriction (caution with hypertensive patients)

- There are two classes of decongestants:
  - o Indirect action sympathomimetics: cause presynaptic release of norepinephrine, which attaches to α_2, presynaptic and α_1 postsynaptic adrenergic receptors, as well as weakly attaching to β adrenergic receptors (ephedrine, pseudoephedrine)

- o Direct action sympathomimetics: agonists for α_2 presynaptic and α_1 postsynaptic adrenergic receptors (imidazolines) or α_1 postsynaptic only (phenylephrine); the presynaptic link reduces norepinephrine production, which partly explains congestion rebound when stopping after prolonged use

- Not to be used without the consent of a physician in the presence of:

  - o Hyperthyroidism (risk of decompensated thyrotoxicosis)
  - o Diabetes (possible glycemic imbalance)
  - o Ischemic cardiovascular diseases (dose-related increase in heart rate)
  - o Hypertension (dose-related increase in blood pressure; effect related to the peak in blood concentration, thus, if indicated, choose sustained release)
  - o Heart failure (post-loading increase; increase in heart rate is a risk for arrhythmias)
  - o Angle-closure glaucoma
  - o Benign prostatic hyperplasia

- Excessive use can have side effects for the CNS, especially in children and the elderly (tremors, anxiety, insomnia, irritability; more common in children and the elderly)

- There are oral and topical forms of decongestants (nasal spray/drops)

- <u>Oral</u>

  - o More effective because of better absorption, but oral forms have a greater number of systemic effects (warning: side effects and interactions)
  - o Less rapid onset of action (compared with spray)
  - o Longer acting (compared with spray) (except xylometazoline and oxymetazoline, the effects of which last up to 12 hours)

- <u>Spray</u>

  - o More practical, especially with adults

- <u>Drops</u>
  - ○ Recommended for children under 6 years
- Topical decongestants should be used no more than 3–5 consecutive days to avoid rebound nasal congestion when treatment stops (*Rhinitis medicamentosa*)

Table II: Treating Rebound Effect of Topical Decongestants
· Stop use in one nostril and continue use in the other
· When rebound effect disappears in the nostril without medication, stop product use entirely
· Use oral decongestants or saline solutions prn

Table III: Oral Decongestants

Medication	Adult Dosage	Side Effects	Interactions	Contraindications/Warnings
Pseudoephedrine	30–60 mg q4–6h or 120 mg of sustained release formulation q12h Maximum 240 mg/day	• CNS stimulation (nervousness, insomnia, excitability, dizziness) • Increase in blood pressure	• MAOIs: hypertensive crisis	• Patients with cardiovascular disease • Hypertension • Hyperthyroidism • Diabetes • Angle-closure glaucoma • Benign prostatic hyperplasia ⇨ Refer to a physician
Phenylephrine	10 mg q4h	• Tachycardia/palpitations • Can affect glycemia in diabetics		

Table IV: Topical Decongestants

Medication	Adult Dosage	Side Effects	Duration of Action
Phenylephrine	Solutions 0.25–0.5% • 1–2 drops/spray q4h in each nostril	• Tingling/localized burning • Sneezing • Nasal dryness • Rebound effect (with > 3 days consecutive use) • Brady/tachycardia and hypo/hypertension have been reported	≈ 4 hours
Naphazoline	Solutions 0.05% • 1–2 drops q6h		≈ 4–6 hours
Oxymetazoline	Solutions 0.05% • 2–3 drops/spray q12h		≈ 12 hours
Xylometazoline	Solutions 0.1% • 2–3 drops/spray q8–10h		≈ 12 hours

Cough

- If cold-related, will last < 2 weeks
- If it lasts > 2 weeks, see a physician
- Camphor, menthol, eucalyptus: effective as topical agents
- Dextromethorphan: for soothing non-productive cough but not for chronic or persistent cough

Table V: Antitussives/Expectorants			
Medication	**Adult Dosage**	**Side Effects**	**Interactions**
Dextromethorphan (DM)	30 mg q6–8h Max.:120 mg/day Onset of action: • 15–30 minutes	• Well tolerated • Nausea • Drowsiness	• MAOIs • SSRIs (especially with paroxetine and fluoxetine) • CYP2D6 inhibitors
Codeine	10–20 mg q4–6h Max. 120 mg/day (8–15 mg codeine has about same antitussive effect as DM 15–30 mg) Onset of action: • 1–2 h	• Drowsiness • Sedation • Nausea/vomiting • Dry mouth • Constipation	• CNS depressants (other opiates, tricyclic antidepressants, alcohol, phenothiazines)
Guaifenesin (expectorant)	200–400 mg q4h Max. 2.4 g/day	• Rare • Nausea/Vomiting • Drowsiness	

Fever

- Three OTC products: ASA/acetaminophen/ibuprofen
- ASA: contraindicated for children (< 18 years), because of possibility of Reye's syndrome
- Acetaminophen: often first choice
- ASA/ibuprofen: anti-inflammatory effect

Allergic rhinitis

- Most effective treatment is to limit exposure to allergens
- Anti-H_1 first generation: + sedative, possible paradoxical effect in children

Table VI: Antihistamines				
Medication	**Adult Dosage**	**CNS**	**Anti-ACh**	**GI**
Anti-H_1 first generation				
Brompheniramine	4–8 mg q4–8h 8–12 mg sustained release q12–24h	+	++	-
Chlorpheniramine	4 mg q4–6h or 8–12 mg sustained release q6–8h Max.: 24 mg/day	+	++	-
Clemastine	1.34–2.68 mg q8–12h Max.: 8.04 mg/day	++	+++	+
Cyproheptadine	4 mg q8–12h Max.: 32 mg/day or 0.5 mg/kg/day	+	++	-
Dexbrompheniramine	2 mg q4–6h SR: 6 mg q12h Max.: 12 mg/day	+	++	-
Diphenhydramine	25–50 mg q4–6h Max.: 300 mg/day	++	+++	+
Doxylamine	7.5–12.5 mg q4–6h Max.: 75 mg/day	++	+++	?
Triprolidine	2.5 mg q6h	+	++	-

Table VI: Antihistamines (cont'd)					
Medication	**Adult Dosage**	**CNS**	**Anti-ACh**	**GI**	**Comments**
Anti-H₁ second generation					
Cetirizine	5–10 mg qd Max.: 10 mg/day	+/-	+/-	+	• Active metabolite of hydroxyzine • If Clcr < 30 mL/min or hepatic failure: 5 mg qd
Fexofenadine	60 mg q12h or 120 mg sustained release q24h Max.: 180 mg/day	+/-	+/-	-	• First choice > 12 years
Loratadine	10 mg qd Max.: 10 mg/day	+/-	+/-	+	• If Clcr < 30 mL/min or hepatic failure: administer dose q48h • First choice < 12 years
Desloratadine	5 mg qd Max.: 5 mg/day	+/-	+/-	+	
Membrane Stabilizers					
Sodium cromoglycate	2–4 spray 3–6 times /day				• Take 2 weeks before exposure

When to consult

- Severe and persistent symptoms (> 7 days)
- Suspected secondary bacterial infections
- Patient who could benefit from a vaccination or a viral neuraminidase inhibitor
- Prolonged fever (> 3 days) or severe fever(> 40°C)
- Presence of dyspnea, change and/or increase in expectoration

References

- Bisno AL. Acute Pharyngitis. N Engl J Med. 2001; 344:205-11.
- Brock TP, Williams DM. Acute and chronic rhinitis. In: Koda-Kimble MA, Young LY, Kradjan WA, Guglielmo BJ. Applied therapeutics: the clinical use of drugs. 8th edition, Philadelphia: Lippincott Williams & Wilkins; 2005. p. 25-1-25-32.
- Covington TR. Nonprescription drug therapy: guiding patient self-care. 2nd edition. St. Louis: Facts & Comparisons; 2003. p. 1302.
- Dicpinigaitis PV. Angiotensin-converting enzyme inhibitor-induced cough: ACCP evidence-based clinical practice guidelines. CHEST. 2006; 129:S169-73.
- Ebell MH, Smith MA, Barry HC, Ives K, Carey M. Does this patient have strep throat? JAMA. 2000; 284:2912-18.
- Heikkinen T, Järvinen A. The common cold. Lancet. 003; 361: 51-9.
- Hoffman BB. Adrenoceptor-activating & other sympathomimetic drugs. In: Basic and clinical pharmacology. 10th edition. New York: McGraw-Hill; 2007. p. 121-40.
- Anonymous. MMWR. 2004; 53; 923-4.
- Monto AS, Gravenstein S, Elliott M, Colopy M, Schweinle J. Clinical signs and symptoms predicting influenza infection. Arch Intern Med. 2000; 160:3245-7.
- Nicholson KG, Wood JM, Zambon M. Influenza. Lancet. 2003; 362: 1733-45.
- Piccirillo JF. Acute bacterial sinusitis. N Engl J Med. 2004; 351: 902-10.
- Ramey JT, Bailen E, Lockey RF. Rhinitis Medicamentosa. J Investig Allergol Clin Immunol. 2006;16:148-55.
- Roy H. Allergic rhinitis. In: Repchinsky C, Leblanc C, editors. Patient self-care: helping patients make therapeutic choices. 1st edition. Ottawa: Canadian Pharmacists Association; Welcom Ltd: 2002. p. 117-29.
- Roy H. Upper respiratory tract infections. In: Repchinsky C, Leblanc C, editors. Patient self-care: helping patients make therapeutic choices. 1st edition. Ottawa: Canadian Pharmacists Association; Welcom Ltd: 2002. p. 130-42.
- Salerno SM, Jackson JL, Berbano EP. Effect of oral pseudoephedrine on blood pressure and heart rate: a meta-analysis. Arch Intern Med. 2005; 165:1686-94.
- Simons FER. Advances in H1-Antihistamines. N Engl J Med. 2004; 351:2203-17.
- Plaut M, Valentine MD. Allergic rhinitis. N Engl J Med. 2005; 353: 1934-44.
- Pratter MR, Brightling CE, Boulet LP, Irwin RS. An empiric integrative approach to the management of cough: ACCP evidence-based clinical practice guidelines. CHEST. 2006; 129: S222-31.
- Tietze KJ. Disorders related to cold and allergy. In: Berardi RR. Handbook of nonprescription drugs: an interactive approach to self-care. 14th edition., Washington: American Pharmacists Association; 2004. p. 239-69.

Pain

Pain

Questions to ask

✓ **Location of pain?**

✓ **Description of pain:**

- o Somatic—evaluate
  - – Relatively well localized
  - – Increases with movement
  - – Constant, deep, bothersome
- o Visceral—refer to a physician
  - – Not clearly defined—difficult to pinpoint location
  - – Accompanied by nausea, vomiting
  - – Related to specific cutaneous sites with skin sensitivity
- o Neuropathic—refer to a physician
  - – Burning sensation (shooting/sharp pain, persistent throbbing pain, electric shocks, stabbing pain)
  - – Localized along nerve paths
  - – Difficult to relieve

✓ **Intensity of pain? (a scale from 1–10 can facilitate evaluation of intensity)**

✓ **For how long?**

✓ **Is the pain acute (short duration) or chronic (long duration)?**

✓ **Has it changed over time? If yes, in what way?**

✓ **What are the exacerbating or relieving factors?**

✓ **Consulted a physician? If yes, what was the diagnosis?**

✓ **What treatments or medications did the physician recommend?**

✓ **To relieve symptoms, what treatments or medications have been tried?**

✓ **Did treatments or medications reduce the pain?**

✓ **If yes, was relief complete or partial?**

✓ **Does the pain affect quality of life?**

✓ **Other medications**

✓ **Medication allergy or intolerance?**

What to do

- If possible, eliminate triggering or exacerbating factors
- Apply hot or cold compresses

HOT or COLD?
Immediately after a trauma: COLD for 24–48 hours
· Reduces pain by inducing local anesthesia
· Decreases internal bleeding and ecchymosis
· Limits edema, distortion, and muscular spasms
· Do not apply ice directly on skin
· Do not apply more than 30 minutes at a time, and wait at least 30 minutes between applications
** N.B.: Contraindications in regard to cold application:
o Raynaud's syndrome: can cause arterial spasms and thus exacerbate disease symptomology
o Arthritis: cold can cause joint stiffness
After 48 hours, when inflammatory reaction has ended, apply HEAT
· Increases local blood circulation
· Reduces joint stiffness, pain, and muscular spasms
· Reduces edema and exudate
· Heat must not be applied directly on the skin
· Do not apply on site of bleeding, thrombophlebitis, or counterirritants

RICE Principle
· **R**est
· **I**ce: Apply cold for 20 minutes 3–4 times/day for 24–48 hours, then apply heat
· **C**ompression: cold toes or fingers indicate bandage too tight
· **E**levation: elevate limb above the heart in order to reduce swelling

What to use

Table I: Dosage and Characteristics of Oral Analgesics		
Analgesic	**Dosage**	**Characteristic(s)**
Acetaminophen (e.g., *Tylenol*)	<u>Adults:</u> 325–1000 mg q4–6h prn (max. 4 g/day) <u>Children:</u> 10–15 mg/kg/dose q4–6h prn (max. 5 doses/day)	Warning: hepatic failure
Ibuprofen (e.g., *Motrin* or *Advil*)	<u>Adults:</u> 200–400 mg q4–6h prn (max.1.2 g qd in self-medication) <u>Children > 6 months:</u> 5–10 mg/kg/dose q6–8h prn (max. 40 mg/kg/day)	Take with food Warning: history of gastric ulcers, renal failure, hypertension, anti-coagulation
Codeine	<u>Adults:</u> 15–60 mg q4–6h prn <u>Children:</u> 0.5–1 mg/kg q4–6h prn Max.: 60 mg/dose	Possibility of cross-allergy with morphine Side effects: Drowsiness, dizziness, nausea, vomiting, constipation, dependence
Caffeine	At least 65 mg in association with acetaminophen or ASA (also depends on patient's daily coffee consumption)	In combination: decreases action onset time and increases analgesic effect Psychomotor stimulation: can cause insomnia

- **Topical analgesics**
  - Generally safe and well tolerated
  - Their use during thermotherapy is not advised because of increased risk of burns

Table II: Dosage and Characteristics of Topical Analgesics		
Analgesic	**Ingredient(s)**	**Characteristic(s)**
Counterirritants with a cooling sensation	Camphor 3–11% Eucalyptus oil 0.5–3% Menthol 1.25–16%	Characteristic odour
Counterirritants that generate warmth	Capsaicin 0.025–0.25%	Burning sensation that eventually disappears with substance P depletion Useful for neuropathic pain Dosage: 1 local application 3–4 times/day over 4–6 weeks
	Methyl salicylate 10–60%	Avoid if patient is allergic to salicylates and with anticoagulated patients (possible systemic absorption)
Salicylates	Triethanolamine salicylate 10–20%	Odourless when moderate massage Avoid if patient is allergic to salicylates and with anticoagulated patients

- **If pain is muscular**
  - **Myorelaxants:** recommended as **second-line** agents; analgesics remain the first choice for treatment
  - Currently, no evidence to suggest that combining ibuprofen with a muscle relaxant increases treatment efficacy

Table III: Dosage and Characteristics of Muscle Relaxants		
Agent	**Dosage**	**Characteristic(s)**
Methocarbamol (e.g., *Robaxin*)	<u>Adults</u>: 1–1.5 g q6h prn (max. 6–8 g/day x 48–72h, then 4 g/day) <u>Children</u>: Not indicated	Short-term use only (x 2–3 days) Can cause drowsiness, blurred vision, dizziness Available alone or with acetaminophen, ibuprofen, or ASA
Orphenadrine (e.g., *Norflex*)	<u>Adults</u>: 25–50 mg q6–8h (max. 200 mg/day) <u>Children</u>: Not indicated	Short-term use only (x 2–3 days) Can cause drowsiness and have anticholinergic effects. Available alone (*Norflex*) or with ASA and caffeine (*Norgesic*)
Chlorzoxazone *available only in combination with acetaminophen* (e.g., *Parafon*)	<u>Adults</u>: 250–500 mg q6–8h (max. 3 g/day) <u>Children</u>: 20 mg/kg/day in 3–4 divided doses	Short-term use only (x 2–3 days) Can cause drowsiness, blurred vision, dizziness, orange-reddish urine Cases of hepatotoxicity Available with acetaminophen

When to consult

- Visceral pain

- Neuropathic pain

- Suspected fracture

- Evidence of joint deformations

- Immobilization for more than 24 hours without symptom improvement

- Pain not relieved by adequate self-medication of more than 14 days for sports injuries or 3–4 weeks for back pain

References

- Desmarais N. Les relaxants musculaires. Québec Pharmacie. 2005; 52:17-21.
- Kissick J. Sports injuries. In: Gray J, editor. Therapeutic choices. 2nd edition. Ottawa: Canadian Pharmacists Association; 2003. p. 647-54.
- Kwan D, Papoushek C. Low back pain. In: Repchinsky C, Leblanc C, editors. Patient self-care: helping patients make therapeutic choices. 1st edition. Ottawa: Canadian Pharmacists Association; Welcom Ltd: 2002. p. 415-25.
- Lum L. Sports injuries. In: Repchinsky C, Leblanc C, editors. Patient self-care: helping patients make therapeutic choices. 1st edition. Ottawa: Canadian Pharmacists Association; Welcom Ltd: 2002. p. 439-46.
- Potvin C. Les analgésiques externes: comment choisir? Québec Pharmacie. 2001; 48:292-94.
- Tunks E. Low back pain. In: Gray J. editor. Therapeutic choices; 2nd edition. Ottawa: Canadian Pharmacists Association; 2003. 589-98.
- Valtonen EJ. A double-blind trial of methocarbamol versus placebo in painful muscle spasm. Curr Med Res Opin. 1975; 3:382-5.
- Watson CP, Tyler KL, Bickers DR, Millikan LE, Smith S, Coleman E. A randomized vehicle-controlled trial of topical capsaicin in the treatment of postherpetic neuralgia. Clin Ther. 1993;15:510-26.

Women's Health

Dysmenorrhea

Dysmenorrhea

Overview

- Painful menstruation that takes place during the ovulatory cycle, not related to any underlying pelvic pathology. Dysmenorrhea is caused by frequent prolonged uterine contractions induced by prostaglandins which decrease the blood flow to the myometrium, resulting in ischemia

- Often begins in adolescence
  - Frequent: occurs in 60–70% of young women

- Risk factors: being under 30 years of age, body mass index under 20, menarche before age 12, prolonged, heavy menstrual cycle, intense bleeding, premenstrual syndrome/depression, cigarette smoking, and pelvic inflammatory disease

Questions to ask

✓ **What are the perceived symptoms and how long have they been present?**

- Symptoms of dysmenorrhea: recurring cramps in the suprapubic region that may radiate to the back and pelvis, headache, fatigue, nausea, vomiting, diarrhea, nervousness, dizziness, and, in some cases, syncope. Symptoms usually appear about 12 hours before menstrual flow begins and become more severe for 7–24 hours, then continue on average for 24–72 hours

- Usually appear 6–12 months after menarche, when ovulatory cycles are well established

- Characteristics of menstruation: regular cycles, the year of menarche (if a young girl)

✓ **History of pelvic disease: endometriosis, adenomyosis, uterine polyps, polycystic ovary disease**

✓ **Patient's age?**

✓ **Age of menarche and when pain first appeared?**

✓ **Duration of menstrual cycle?**

✓ **Impact of pain on daily activities?**

✓ **Agents already used for menstrual cramps and their efficacy?**

✓ **History of gastroduodenal ulcer?**

✓ **Other medications taken concomitantly?**

What to do

- Physical exercise increases blood flow in the pelvic area and helps to ease symptoms

- Stop smoking: the incidence of dysmenorrhea is higher among smokers

- Adopt a diet low in fat, and increase intake of omega-3 polyunsaturated fatty acids

- Hot-water bottle placed on the abdomen (as effective as taking oral medication)

- Relaxation (yoga, low-impact exercise, hot bath, etc.)

What to use

- Ibuprofen is the treatment of choice in over-the-counter products

- Pharmacological treatment (NSAIDs) must be started early, at the beginning of the menstrual cycle
  - The trial period is 3 months. In the event of insufficient efficacy, you may consider increasing the dosage or changing agents

- Hormonal contraception under prescription is also an option to be considered if needed (second-line drug therapy)
  - Trial period of 3 months
  - Should contain 20–35 µg of estrogen

- For patients who respond well to the agent, it is not necessary to begin medication before the first day of the menstrual cycle. On the other hand, it is recommended that the medication be taken regularly rather than on an as needed basis

Table I: Drug Therapy for Dysmenorrhea		
Agent	**Dosage**	**Comments**
Ibuprofen (*Motrin, Advil*)	200–400 mg q4–6h Max: 1.2 g/day for OTC treatment Under prescription, may go to 800 mg as freely as wanted q6h	First choice of OTC treatment Take with food
Acetylsalicylic acid (*Aspirin, Entrophen, Bufferin*)	500–650 mg q4–6h Max: 3.6 g/day	Less effective than other NSAIDs
Acetaminophen (*Tylenol, Atasol*)	325–650 mg q4–6h Max: 4 g/day	Has no anti-inflammatory effect Use if NSAIDs or ASA are contraindicated or not effective
Muscle relaxants Methocarbamol Orphenadrine	In compounds combined with an NSAID, ASA, or with acetaminophen	Few data supporting their efficacy
Diuretics Pamabron Caffeine		
Antihistamines Pyrilamine Maleate Doxylamine Succinate		
Magnesium	Many dosages under study No optimal dosage determined	More effective than placebo in some randomized studies (However, studies contain many biases)
Hormonal contraceptives may be an interesting option if the patient wants contraception		

- Thiamine, Vitamin E, and omega-3 fatty acids have all been studied for dysmenorrhea and could be effective according to randomized studies

When to consult

- History of pelvic disease: endometriosis, adenomyosis, uterine polyps, or polycystic ovary disease
- Non-classical symptoms
- Inefficacy of OTCs
- Contraindications for OTCs
- Inefficacy of hormonal contraceptives after a trial period of 3–6 months

References

- Doty E , Arraran M. Managing primary dysmenorrhea. J Pediatr Adolesc Gynecol. 2006; 19: 341-4.
- French L. Dysmenorrhea. American Family Physician. 2005; 71: 285-291.
- Fankhauser MP. Menstrual-related disorders. In: Di Piro JT, Talbert RL, Yee GC, Matzke GR, Wells BG, Posey LM, editors. Pharmacotherapy: a pathophysiology approach. 4th edition. United States: McGraw-Hill Companies; 1999. p. 1349-50.
- Gill GH. Dysmenorrhea. In: Gray J, editor. Therapeutic choices. 3rd edition. Ottawa: Canadian Pharmacists Association; 2000. p. 578-83.
- Harel Z. Dysmenorrhea in adolescents and young adults: etiology and management. J Pediatr Adolesc Gynecol. 2006; 19: 363-371.
- Pray SW. Consult your pharmacist–dysmenorrhea: how to relieve cramps. [Internet]. Us Pharmacist 2000. [cited 2007 May 20]. Available from:. http://www.medscape.com/view article/407634
- Proctor M, Farquhar C. Diagnosis and management of dysmenorrhoea. BMJ. 2006; 332: 1134-8.
- Smith RP et Barbieri RL. Treatment of primary dysmenorrhea in adult women. [Internet]. UpToDate Online. [cited 2007 May 20]. Available from:http://www.uptodate.com.

Emergency Contraception

Emergency Contraception

This chapter is a memory aid and is not intended to replace training or professional experience or a rigorous review of the principles for prescribing emergency contraception (EC). Given the topic in question, it is all the more important to take a comprehensive personalized approach.

<u>Questions to ask</u>

✓ **Reason for the consultation**

✓ **Patient's age (must be over 14 years of age)**

✓ **Type of sexual intercourse risk**

- o Unprotected sex

- o Failure of barrier method (condom)

- o Late by 2 or more oral contraceptive pills, or 2 or more pills forgotten

- o One week or more late with *Depo-Provera* injection

- o Interrupted coitus

- o Preventive measure in case of travel, treatment with *Accutane*

✓ **Date and time of risky sexual intercourse**

✓ **Risky sexual intercourse in the past 7 days**

✓ **Contraception used**

✓ **Date of last menstrual period**

✓ **Length of menstrual cycle**

✓ **Character of menstruation flow (normal or abnormal)**

✓ **Risk of sexually transmitted disease**

✓ **Risk of sexual intercourse being the result of sexual assault**

What to do

- Get the consent of a parent or guardian (in accordance with the Civil Code) if the patient is under 14 years of age (exceptions apart)

- Advise youth protection services if sexual assault is suspected in the case of a patient under 18

- Suggest a pregnancy test if:

    o the last menstrual period was more than 28 days ago

    o menstrual bleeding did not resume 21 days after taking EC

    o The last menstrual period was abnormal (quantity and/or duration)

    o Pregnancy is suspected

What to use

- Within 72 hours of risky sexual intercourse:

    o **Yuzpe method**
        - *Ovral* 2 tablets q12h x 2 doses
          + 25–50 mg Gravol 30–60 minutes predose prn

Table I: Ovral Equivalent Doses		
Oral contraceptive	**Number of tablets per dose**	**EE (µg)/LNG (µg)**
Ovral	2	100/500
Alesse	5	100/500
Triquilar	4 yellow tablets	120/500
Minovral	4 yellow tablets	120/600

EE: ethynylestradiol   LNG: levonorgestrel

Adapted from the Ordre des pharmaciens du Québec and from the Ministère de la Santé et des Services Sociaux du Québec. La contraception orale d'urgence : Manuel d'auto-information à l'intention des pharmaciennes et des pharmaciens. January 2002.

- The most frequent side effects when the usual contraceptive pills are used for emergency contraception are:
    - Nausea (30–60%)
    - Vomiting (12–22%)

- Dizziness
- Fatigue
- Breast tenderness
- Headache

o **Levonorgestrel alone**
- *Plan B*: 1 tablet q12h x 2 doses or 2 tablets x 1 dose
- Administration of a double dose of 1.5 mg of levonorgestrel (2 tablets) seems as effective as administration in 2 doses. This option may be considered when the dosing interval may not be observed
- First choice if:
  - Breastfeeding
  - Nausea, vomiting, migraine
  - Treatment with an antibiotic
  - Treatment with warfarin
  - History of stroke
- Side effects are less frequent with *Plan B* than with combined oral contraceptives [e.g., nausea (23%), vomiting (6%)]

- The efficacy of EC varies depending on the delay between taking the medication and unprotected sexual intercourse

- The earlier the dose is taken after unprotected sex, the greater the efficacy

  o According to some studies, the efficacy of EC may extend up to 120 hours after unprotected sex

  o The failure rate for the Yuzpe method after a delay of 72 hours is 4% (pregnancies), compared with 10% after 120 hours

- In the event of vomiting less than an hour after taking the EC pill, it is necessary to take the drug again. Taking an antiemetic is also advised

- Menstruation should appear within 21 days of taking the last EC pill (occurring in 98% of patients)

- If EC is taken before ovulation, menstrual bleeding should appear 3–7 days earlier

- In 90% of patients, menstrual flow and duration were normal after taking EC
- EC is not a contraceptive method
- <u>When to begin regular contraception</u>
  - As soon as sexual intercourse resumes, with regard to **barrier methods**
  - Within the first 7 days of the menstrual cycle for *Depo-Provera*, with a barrier method until menstruation begins
  - **Oral hormonal contraception**
    - New pill pack the very next day, plus barrier method for 7 days including the day EC was taken, or
    - Barrier method until next menstrual cycle. Then start a new pill pack
    - Pregnancy test recommended if no menstruation occurs 28 days after resumption of oral hormonal contraceptives

When to consult

- Patients under 14 years of age
- Emergency contraception period has passed (an IUD may be used up to 7 days after unprotected sex)
- Positive pregnancy test
- The patient wants to begin a hormonal contraception method on a regular basis
- Detection of STD or HIV
- Suspicion of sexual assault or abuse (referral to hospital Emergency Room for an evidence kit is required)

References

- Canadian Pharmacists Association. Compendium of nonprescription products. 38th edition. Ottawa: Canadian Pharmacists Association, 2003.
- Cheng L, Gulmezoglu AM, Oel CJ, Piaggio G, Ezcurra E, Look PF. Interventions for emergency contraception. Cochrane Database SystRev. 2004; 3: CD001324. Review.
- Dunn S, Guilbert E, Lefebvre G, et al. Clinical practice gynaecology and social sexual issues committees, Society of Obstetricians and Gynaecologists of Canada (SOGC). Emergency contraception. J Obstet Gynaecol Can. 2003; 25: 673-9, 680-7; quiz 688-90.
- Ellertson C. Emergency contraception: a review of the programmatic and social science literature contraception. Contraception. 2000; 61: 145-86.
- Hasen LB, Saseen JJ, Teal SB. Levonorgestrel-only dosing strategies for emergency contraception. Pharmacotherapy. 2007; 27: 278-84.
- Ordre des pharmaciens du Québec et Santé et Services sociaux du Québec. La contraception orale d'urgence: manuel d'auto-information à l'intention des pharmaciennes et des pharmaciens. January 2002. Quebec: Ordre des pharmaciens du Québec.
- Canadian Paediatric Society (CPS). Emergency contraception. Paediatrics & Child Health. 2003; 8 (3):181-183.
- Task Force on Postovulatory Methods of Fertility Regulation. Randomised controlled trial of levonorgestrel versus the Yuzpe regimen of combined oral contraceptives for emergency contraception. Lancet.1998; 352:428-33.
- Weismiller DG.Emergency contraception. Am Fam Physician. 2004; 70: 707-14.

Missed Hormonal Contraceptive

Missed Hormonal Contraceptive

Questions to ask

- ✓ **What hormonal contraceptive is being used?**
- ✓ **On what date was the pill pack started?**
- ✓ **How many tablets were missed?**
- ✓ **When was the last time unprotected sex took place?**
- ✓ **When was last menstrual period?**

What to do

Combined oral contraceptives, including *Yasmin* (except *Diane-35*)

WHEN THE CYCLE BEGINS ON A SUNDAY

- **When 1 pill was missed**
  - o Take the pill as soon as possible. The patient might therefore have to take 2 pills the same day
- **When 2 consecutive pills were missed**

  Under the first two weeks of the pill pack

  - o Take 2 pills the day it is realized that pills were missed, and 2 pills the next day
  - o Continue taking pills regularly, 1 pill a day until all pills in the pack have been taken

<u>During the third week of the pill pack</u>

- o Take 1 pill a day until the upcoming Sunday
- o That Sunday, discard the rest of the pill pack and begin a new one
- o There may not be menstruation that month

- **When 3 consecutive pills were missed, regardless of when in the cycle**
    - o Take 1 pill a day until the upcoming Sunday
    - o That Sunday, discard the rest of the pill pack and begin a new one
    - o There may be an absence of menstruation that month

WHEN THE CYCLE BEGINS ON A DAY OTHER THAN SUNDAY

- **When 1 pill was missed**
    - o Take the pill as soon as possible. The patient might therefore have to take 2 pills the same day

- **When 2 consecutive pills were missed**
    <u>During the first two weeks of the pill pack</u>
    - o Take 2 pills the day it is realized that pills were missed, and 2 pills the next day
    - o Continue taking pills regularly, 1 pill a day until all pills in the pack have been taken

    <u>During the third week of the pill pack</u>
    - o The day it is realized that a pill was missed, discard the rest of the pill pack and begin a new one the very same day

- **When 3 consecutive pills were missed, regardless of when in the cycle**
    - o The day it is realized that a pill has been missed, discard the rest of the pill pack and begin a new one the very same day

---

If 2 or more pills were missed, regardless of the first day of the cycle, recommend a back-up contraceptive method during sexual intercourse for at least 7 days after the pills were missed

---

Table I: Steps to Follow after Missed Pill

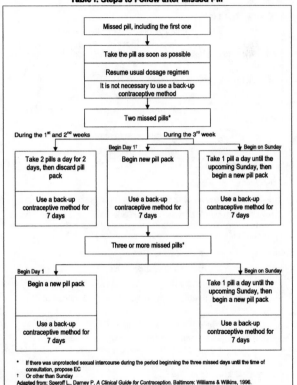

Missed pill, including the first one

↓

Take the pill as soon as possible

↓

Resume usual dosage regimen

↓

It is not necessary to use a back-up contraceptive method

↓

Two missed pills*

During the 1ˢᵗ and 2ⁿᵈ weeks | **During the 3ʳᵈ week**

Begin Day 1† | Begin on Sunday

Take 2 pills a day for 2 days, then discard pill pack	Begin new pill pack	Take 1 pill a day until the upcoming Sunday, then begin a new pill pack
Use a back-up contraceptive method for 7 days	Use a back-up contraceptive method for 7 days	Use a back-up contraceptive method for 7 days

↓

Three or more missed pills*

Begin Day 1 | Begin on Sunday

Begin a new pill pack	Take 1 pill a day until the upcoming Sunday, then begin a new pill pack
Use a back-up contraceptive method for 7 days	Use a back-up contraceptive method for 7 days

* If there was unprotected sexual intercourse during the period beginning the three missed days until the time of consultation, propose EC

† Or other than Sunday

Adapted from: Speroff L., Darney P. *A Clinical Guide for Contraception*. Baltimore: Williams & Wilkins, 1996.

Diane-35

- **If < 12 hours late**
  - The patient must take the pill as soon as possible
  - The patient must then continue taking pills at the usual time of day. The patient might therefore have to take 2 pills the same day

- **If > 12 hours late**
  - The patient must discard the missed pill
  - The patient must then continue taking pills at the usual time of day
  - A back-up method of contraception must be used until all the pills in the pack have been taken

Contraceptive patch (*Evra*)

DURING WEEK 1 OF THE CYCLE

- Use a back-up contraceptive method for 1 week

- Apply a new patch as soon as the patient remembers. She will then have a new patch change day and will have to apply the next patch one week later (not on her usual day)

DURING WEEK 2 OR 3 OF THE CYCLE

- **If the patch is changed 1 or 2 days late**
  - Remove the used patch and apply a new one immediately
  - The following patch must be applied on the usual patch change day
  - No back-up contraceptive method is necessary

- With the *Evra* contraceptive patch, targeted hormonal concentrations are maintained for 9 days following 1 complete cycle

- **If more than 2 days late**
  - If there was sexual intercourse during this period, use of emergency contraception (EC) may be considered

- o Use a back-up contraceptive method for 1 week
- o The used patch is removed and a new one applied as soon as the patient remembers, then a new 4-week cycle is begun
- o The patch change day will no longer be the same

DURING WEEK 4 OF THE CYCLE

- The patient must remove the patch as soon as she remembers
- Begin the cycle following the usual patch change day
- No back-up contraceptive method is necessary if the period from the moment the patch is removed until a new one is applied is under 7 days

IF THE PATCH BECOMES DETACHED

- **Within 24 hours**
  - o Remove the patch and immediately apply a new one
  - o No back-up contraceptive method is necessary
  - o The patch change day stays the same
- **After more than 24 hours or after an unknown lapse of time**
  - o If there was sexual intercourse, EC should be considered
  - o Start a new 4-week cycle
  - o The cycle change day will no longer be the same
  - o Use a back-up contraceptive method during the first week of the new cycle

Contraceptive vaginal ring (*Nuvaring*)

- **If the ring is accidentally expelled or removed from the vagina for less than 3 hours**
  - o Rinse the ring and reinsert it
  - o No other contraceptive method is necessary

- **If the ring is accidentally expelled and is left outside of the vagina for more than 3 continuous hours or if no ring has been used for 7 days**
  - Another contraceptive method will be necessary for 7 days
- **If the ring has been in the vagina for a prolonged period; more than 3 weeks but less than 4 weeks**
  - Protection against possible pregnancy is maintained
  - No other contraceptive method is necessary
- **If the ring has been in the vagina for more than 4 weeks**
  - Remove the ring
  - Consider EC because protection may be inadequate
  - Wait one week, then insert a new ring

Progestin-only oral contraceptives (*Micronor*/*Depo-Provera*)

Oral contraceptives (*Micronor*)

A *Micronor* pack contains 28 active tablets

- **If 1 pill missed or > 3 hours late**
  - The missed pill should be taken as soon as possible
  - The patient should then continue taking the remaining pills at the usual time of day. The patient might therefore have to take 2 pills the same day
  - Use a back-up contraceptive method for 48 hours after the missed pill
  - There may be spotting, even if the missed dose was taken as soon as remembered

Depo-Provera Intramuscular injections

- If the last injection was less than 14 weeks ago (late by 2 weeks or less), the next injection can be administered

What to use

- EC if indications are met (see below)
- Pregnancy test if the date of the last menstrual period was over 4 weeks ago

When to consult

- If no menstrual period 2 months in a row
- If there was unprotected sex during the period beginning 3 days before the missed date
- Indications for prescribing EC, <u>in the event of inadequate use of hormonal contraceptives</u>
  - When 2 or more of the usual oral contraceptive pills were missed, or the patient was more than 2 days late in resuming oral contraceptives
  - When 2 or more weeks late administering *Depo-Provera*

References

- Canadian Pharmacists Association. Compendium of nonprescription products. 38th edition. Ottawa: Canadian Pharmacists Association, 2007.
- Bérubé Jocelyn, et al. Contraception: tour d'horizon et conseils pratiques. Le Médecin du Québec. 2000; 35:89-97.
- Black A, Francoeur D, Rowe T. Canadian Contraception Consensus. Clinical practice guidelines from The Society of Obstetricians and Gynaecologists of Canada. JOGC. 2004; 148: 255-296.
- Carruthers-Czyzewski P, editor. Non-prescription drug reference for health professionals. 1st edition. Ottawa: Canadian Pharmaceutical Association; 1996
- Lacy C, Armstrong LL, Ingrim N, Lance LL. Drug information handbook: a comprehensive resource for all clinicians and healthcare professionals. 14th edition. Hudson: Lexi-Comp Inc; 2006–2007.
- Ordre des pharmaciens du Québec et Santé et Services sociaux du Québec. La contraception orale d'urgence: manuel d'auto-information à l'intention des pharmaciennes et des pharmaciens. January 2002.
- Royal College of Obstetricians and Gynaecologists, UK FFPRHC Guidance (October 2003): First prescription of combined oral contraception. J Fam Plann Reprod Health Care. 2003; 29:209-22.

Osteoporosis

Overview

- Osteoporosis is a systemic skeletal disease characterized by low bone mass and microarchitectural deterioration of bone tissue, with a consequent increase in bone fragility and susceptibility to fracture

- According to the World Health Organization (WHO), the risk of fracture attributable to bone fragility depends both on bone density and on bone architecture

Primary Osteoporosis

- Postmenopausal osteoporosis (type I)
  - Affects women 5–10 years after menopause (Loss of 30–50% of bone mass)
  - Rapid loss of trabecular bone tied to the decrease in circulating estrogen
  - Vertebrae, hip, and wrist bones are the bones most often fractured

- Senile osteoporosis (type II)
  - Age related (elderly over 75 years of age)
  - Present in men and women (1:2)
  - Starting at age 35, bone mass density begins to decrease by 0.3–0.5% a year, in both men and women. This decrease reaches 2–3% in women after menopause
  - Vertebrae, hip, and pelvic bones are the bones most often fractured
  - Calcium deficiency

Secondary Osteoporosis

- Related to the use of medications or to other diseases

- In men and women both (1:1)

Table I: Risk Factors for Osteoporosis			
Genetic factors	**Lifestyle**	**Medications or Drugs**	**Physiological Disorders**
· Caucasian or Asian origin · Family history · Premature menopause · Delayed menstruation · Nulliparity · Low body mass · Small bones · Amenorrhea	· Smoking · Alcohol · Sedentary lifestyle · Low calcium and vitamin D intake · Caffeine · High protein and sodium intake in food · Prolonged immobilization	· Glucocorticoids (>3 months) ≥2.5 mg prednisone/day or equivalent · Levothyroxine in excessive doses · Lithium · Anticonvulsants (phenytoin or phenobarbital) · Cyclosporine · Loop diuretics · Chemotherapy · Long-term treatment with heparin · Proton pump inhibitors ($\downarrow$ absorption of Ca^{2+}) · Excessive use of antacids containing Al^{2+}	· Hyperthyroidism · Primary hyperparathyroidism · Cushing's syndrome · Anorexia · Bulimia · Malabsorption · Prolonged parenteral nutrition · Type I diabetes · Rheumatoid arthritis · Pernicious anemia

What to do

- Change lifestyle habits (smoking, alcohol, diet, exercise)

- Calcium intake in diet, and exercise are the two key elements for preventing osteoporosis

- **Exercise**
  - Physical exercise has a beneficial effect on bone mass. To prevent osteoporosis, stretching exercises are recommended to bring about a correction in posture. Light aerobic exercise and impact exercise are also beneficial

- **Calcium**

Table II: Recommended Calcium Intake	
Age	**Daily Intake (mg)**
4–8 years	800
9–18 years	1300
Premenopausal women	1000
Men < 50 years	1000
Postmenopausal women	1500
Men > 50 years	1500
Women > 18 years pregnant or breastfeeding	1000

Table III: Calcium Content of Some Foods		
Food	**Portion**	**Elemental Calcium (mg)**
Milk (skim)	250 mL	350–450
Milk (whole)	250 mL	250–350
Ice cream	250 mL	200
Cheese (Swiss, gruyère)	50 g	493
Cheese (brick, cheddar, gouda)	50 g	353
Cheese (mozzarella)	50 g	269
Cottage cheese or cream cheese	50 g	87
Yogourt (natural)	175 g	345
Sardines	55 g	210
Pink salmon (canned)	213 g	225
Cooked green beans	250 mL	90
White or whole wheat bread	1 slice	25
Spinach	125 mL	110
Broccoli	125 mL	75
Banana	Average	10
Orange	Average	52
Almonds	125 mL	200

What to use

Table IV: Calcium Supplements			
Salt	**% Elemental Calcium**	**Elemental Calcium**	**Comments**
Calcium carbonate	40%	250 mg = 100 mg of Ca^{2+} 300 mg = 120 mg of Ca^{2+} 500 mg = 200 mg of Ca^{2+} 600 mg = 240 mg of Ca^{2+}	• Available in tablets, syrup, or effervescent tablets • Decreases gastric irritation when taken in divided doses with food • Least expensive
Calcium gluconate	9%	650 mg = 60 mg of Ca^{2+}	• Causes less gastric irritation than carbonate
Calcium lactate	13%	650 mg = 84 mg of Ca^{2+}	• Causes less gastric irritation than carbonate
Calcium citrate	21%	250 mg = 100 mg of Ca^{2+}	• Causes less gastric irritation than carbonate

- o Daily doses of calcium over 2 g cannot be taken except in special cases under the supervision of a physician
- o To minimize side effects related to taking calcium, especially gastric irritation, it is recommended to take the doses broken up during the day (max. 500 mg/dose)

- Vitamin D
  - o Under age 50: 400 IU daily
  - o Over age 50: 800 IU daily

- Other
  - o Under prescription, bisphosphonates and selected estrogen receptor modulators may be prescribed as prevention or as osteoporosis treatment (hormone replacement therapy is no longer indicated given the associated increased risk of breast cancer and myocardial infarction)

When to consult

- Fractures associated with osteoporosis

- Risk factors for developing osteoporosis

- Side effects, resistant to regular treatment

References

- 2002 clinical practice guidelines for the diagnosis and the management of osteoporosis in Canada. CMAJ. 2002;167:S1-S34.
- Cheung AM, et al. Prevention of osteoporosis and osteoporotic fractures in postmenopausal women: recommendation statement from the Canadian Task Force on Preventive Health Care. CMAJ. 2004;170:1-7.
- Cloutier I. Prévention et traitement de l'ostéoporose (part 1). Pharmactuel. 2001; 34:104-10.
- Cloutier I. Prévention et traitement de l'ostéoporose (part 2). Pharmactuel. 2001; 34:125-33.
- Greenblatt. Treatment of Postmenopausal Osteoporosis. Pharmacotherapy. 2005; 25:574-84.
- Lalitha Raman-Wilms. Osteoporosis. In: Repchinsky C, Leblanc C, editors. Patient self-care: helping patients make therapeutic choices. 1st edition. Ottawa: Canadian Pharmacists Association; Welcom Ltd: 2002. p. 406-14.
- Lussier S. La prévention et le traitement de l'ostéoporose. Québec Pharmacie. 2003; 50:27-39.
- O'Connell MB, Seaton TL. Osteoporosis and osteomalacia. In: Di Piro JT, Talbert RL, Yee GC, Matzke GR, Wells BG, Posey LM, editors. Pharmacotherapy: a pathophysiology approach. 6th edition. United States: McGraw-Hill Companies; 2005. p. 1645-1668.
- Parent-Stevens L, Sagraves R. Gynecologic and other disorders of women. Dans: Koda-Kimble MA, et al. Applied therapeutics: the clinical use of drugs. 8th edition. Philadelphia: Lippincott William & Wilkins; 2005. p. 48-28-44.
- Rosen, CJ. Postmenopausal osteoporosis. New Eng J of Med. 2005; 353: 595-603.

Vaginal Dryness
Vaginal Dryness

Questions to ask

✓ **What are the symptoms and how long have they been present?**

   ○ Decrease in vaginal lubrication

   ○ Itching, burning, pain, and irritation

   ○ Difficulties during daily activities or during sexual intercourse that could cause dyspareunia

   ○ Post-coital bleeding

   ○ Malodorous vaginal secretions

   ○ Correlation with a specific time in the menstrual cycle

✓ **Patient's age?**

✓ **Experiencing menopause?**

   ○ Vaginal dryness is directly related to estrogen deficiency

✓ **Recent pregnancy?**

   ○ 20% of women suffer from vaginal atrophy four weeks after giving birth

✓ **Breastfeeding?**

✓ **New at taking hormonal contraceptives?**

✓ **Decrease in sexual activity?**

✓ **Using a vaginal douche or a new soap?**

   ○ Sensitivity to chemical agents (soaps/detergents)

✓ **Tobacco?**

   ○ Tobacco increases the metabolism of estrogen

✓ **New medications?**

- o Anticholinergics (antihistamines, tricyclic antidepressants, antipsychotics), oral contraceptives, estrogen receptor antagonists (tamoxifen), or GnRH analog agonists (leuprolide)

What to do

- Avoid using tampons
- Avoid products that may cause sensitivity (e.g., vaginal douches, perfumed products)
- Stop taking (or decrease) medication at the source of the problem (e.g., anticholinergics) with intervention by the treating physician
- Regular sexual activity can help maintain vaginal health
  - o Based on a clinical study, having sexual relations 3 times a month decreased vaginal atrophy, compared with sexual inactivity
  - o Masturbation could help maintain vaginal secretions and vaginal elasticity

What to use

- There are two types of OTC products: moisturizers and lubricants
  - o Lubricants
    - − Temporary measure to be used before sexual intercourse
    - − Short acting
    - − Combination of protective and thickening agents
    - − May decrease sperm motility, hence contraindicated in women trying to conceive
    - − Petroleum-jelly based agents may impair barrier protection of condoms
  - o Moisturizers are likely to be more effective than lubricants
    - − Longer acting than lubricants (moisturization maintained for more than 24 hours)

- *Replens* can decrease sperm motility, hence avoid for women trying to conceive
- According to certain studies, can have efficacy similar to topical estrogens, but does not alter vaginal morphology

Table I: Vaginal Lubricants and Moisturizers		
Agent	Ingredients	Comments
Replens gel (moisturizer)	Glycerin Mineral oil	1 application every 2–3 days
Vagisil intimate lubricant (lubricant)	Water Glycerin Propylene glycol	1 application prn
Gyne-Moistrin gel (lubricant)	Polyglyceryl methacrylate Propylene glycol	1 application prn
K-Y gel (lubricant)	Chlorhexidine Glycerin	1 application prn

- These products can be used for external or internal application, prn
- Topical or oral phytoestrogens can also be used although their efficacy has not been proven. A few examples:
  - Black cohosh (*Cimicifuga racemosa*)
  - Chasteberry (*Vitex agnus-castus*)
  - Dong Quai creams (*Angelica sinensis*)
  - Wild yam cream (*Dioscorea villosa*)

When to consult

- Problem persists despite nonpharmacological methods
- Problem potentially connected to a prescribed drug
- Presence of vaginal lesions

References

- Bachmann G, Santen RJ. Diagnosis and treatment of atrophic vaginitis. [Internet]. UpToDate. [cited 2007 May 21]. Available from: http://www.uptodate.com.
- Greendale GA, Lee NP, Arriola NR. The menopause. Lancet. 1999; 353:571-80.
- Willhite LA, O'Connell BO. Urogenital atrophy: prevention and treatment. Pharmacotherapy. 2001; 21:464-480.
- Van Voorhis BJ. Genitourinary symptoms in the menopausal transition. Am J Med. 2005; 118:475-535.
- Yuksel N. Prise en charge de l'atrophie vaginale. Continuing education lesson by Rogers Media Ltd. Health and finance edition. February 2005.

Vaginitis

Questions to ask

✓ **What are the symptoms and how long have they been present?**
- Change in vaginal discharge (colour, odour, texture, quantity)
- Pruritus, burning sensation, dyspareunia
- Systemic symptoms: fever, shivers, lower abdominal pain, cutaneous rash

✓ **Are there recent changes in the patient's lifestyle?**
- Changes in detergent, soap
- New undergarments, bathing suit
- Medications taken: antibiotics, corticosteroids, immunosuppressors, hormonal contraceptives, estrogen supplements
- Pregnancy
- Obesity
- Frequency of sexual intercourse, unprotected sex
- Changes in diet: ⇑ quantity of carbohydrates

✓ **Are there other underlying pathologies?**
- Diabetes
- HIV/AIDS or immune deficiency
- Incontinence problems

✓ **Is this the patient's first episode of vaginitis? Has she consulted a physician about it?**

✓ **Determine the risk factors for sexually transmitted infections:**
- Unprotected sex
- Multiple partners

Table I: Classification of Vaginitis			
Type	**Infectious Agents**	**Characteristics of Discharge**	**Symptoms**
Bacterial vaginitis (40–50%) * Risk of pre-term labour in pregnant women	Polymicrobial *Gardnerella vaginalis* *Bacteroides non-fragilis* *Mobiluncus* *Mycoplasma hominis* *Peptococci*	· Foul odour (smells like fish) · White to grayish colour · Homogeneous texture · Moderate amount	· 50% of women are asymptomatic · No dyspareunia
Vulvovaginal candidiasis (20–25%)	*Candida albicans* (80–90%) *C. glabrata* *C. tropicalis* Vaginitis of the Candida species, especially non-albican forms are often more difficult to diagnose	· Cottage cheese texture · Moderate amount	**_Candida albicans_:** · Severe pruritus · Itching · Burning (especially during micturition and sexual intercourse) · Occasional pustules · Dyspareunia · Edema, erythema **Non-albicans _Candida_ vaginitis** more often causes irritation and burning rather than pruritus, often without an increase in secretions The appearance of symptoms a few days before menstruation is typical

Table I: Classification of Vaginitis (cont'd)			
Type	Infectious Agents	Characteristics of Discharge	Symptoms
Trichomonas vaginitis (15–20%)	*Trichomonas vaginitis:* STI ⇨ sexual partner must receive treatment	• Increased moisture in the perineal region • Purulent, foamy, abundant discharge • Yellow/green colour	• Can be asymptomatic • Pruritus possible • Dyspareunia • Erythema
Atrophic vaginitis	Caused by hormonal changes (estrogen deficiency)	• Possible discharge present • Spotting	• Dryness • Burning • Petechiae

What to do

- Maintain good vaginal hygiene: clean the perineal region regularly with a mild soap and water (e.g., *Dove*). The vagina is a self-cleaning organ. No special hygiene measure is indicated. Avoid vaginal douches available on the market because they destroy vaginal flora

- After bowel movements, wipe from front to back to avoid contamination by microbes from the anal region

- Avoid perfumed sanitary products including sanitary napkins, tampons, detergents, soaps, and bubble baths

- Wear loose undergarments and clothing. Choose non-synthetic fibres for better ventilation

- Properly control underlying diseases such as diabetes and HIV/AIDS

- These nonpharmacological means are effective in preventing recurrence

What to use

- Only vulvovaginal candidiasis can be treated with OTC products

- Antifungal agents are the treatment of choice for treating vulvovaginal candidiasis with nonprescription drugs. All OTC products have an efficacy of 80%

- Complicated or refractory infections can be the manifestation of underlying pathologies such as diabetes and immunosuppression. As well, non-albicans species of Candida (*Candida glabrata/krusei*) are usually resistant to the usual topical treatment (azole) and can be a cause of refractory infections

- It is recommended that Combipack formats (containing an additional tube of cream for external application) be used. It is equally important to treat both the vulva and the vagina

- Treatments of 3 days or less are indicated for patients presenting with an uncomplicated infection with no history of recurrence, so as to ensure better compliance

- Treatments of 6 days or more must be used if the infection is recurring (more than 4 episodes a year)

- The improvement of symptoms is noticeable 2 or 3 days after the beginning of treatment, but may be delayed in cases of complicated vaginitis (6 days)

- Continue treatment even during menstruation. Avoid using tampons

- Even though clotrimazole and miconazole in topical application are safe during pregnancy, only those patients who previously consulted a physician should be treated. Vaginal tablets inserted manually are the treatment of choice

- Antifungal creams applied topically, externally, can be used by the sexual partner if the partner is suspected of being the cause of reinfection

- Clotrimazole presents less risk of drug interaction than miconazole

- Topical estrogens are used in the treatment of atrophic vaginitis. Topical or oral phytoestrogens can be used, although their efficacy has not yet been proven

Table II: Antifungal Agents in the Treatment of Vulvovaginal Candidiasis			
Antifungal agent	**Form/Strength**	**Dosage**	**Duration of Treatment**
Clotrimazole *(Canesten Clotrimaderm)*	Vaginal cream 1%*	Contents of 1 applicator at bedtime	6 days
	Vaginal cream 2%		3 days
	Vaginal cream 10%		1 day
	Vaginal tablet 500 mg	1 vaginal tablet at bedtime	1 day
	Vaginal tablet 200 mg		3 days
Miconazole *(Monistat Mycatin)*	Vaginal cream* 2%	Contents of 1 applicator at bedtime	7 days
	Vaginal ovule 400 mg	1 vaginal ovule at bedtime	3 days
	Vaginal ovule 1200 mg		1 day
	Vaginal suppository 100 mg	1 vaginal suppository at bedtime	7 days
Tioconazole *(GyneCure)*	Vaginal ointment* 6.5%	Contents of 1 applicator at bedtime	1 day
	Vaginal ovule 300 mg	1 vaginal ovule at bedtime	1 day
	Topical cream 6.5%/vaginal ointment 1%*	Contents of 1 applicator at bedtime	1 day
	Ovule 300 mg/vaginal cream 1%*	1 vaginal ovule at bedtime	1 day
Terconazole Econazole Nystatin	Vaginal creams, tablets, or suppositories, according to the product	1 application at bedtime	Available under prescription only
Fluconazole	Tablet 150 mg	1 dose	Available under prescription only
Nystatin	Vaginal tablet 100,000 IU	1 vaginal tablet at bedtime	14 days

* Can be used for topical external application

Table III: Other Products		
Product	**Dosage**	**Comments**
Boric acid	Intravaginal capsules, 600 mg qd to bid x 14–28 days	Efficacy reported but not recommended for first-line treatment
Gentian violet 1%	As a tincture	Inconvenient to use. Irritating. Stains clothing
Benzocaine 5% Resorcinol 2% (*Vagisil*)	Local application, prn	For symptomatic treatment only Risk of hypersensitivity reaction
Vaginal douche		Not recommended for routine use

When to consult

- First episode of vaginitis or of refractory vaginitis
- Presence of systemic symptoms
- Vaginal bleeding
- Absence of clinical improvement after 3 days or absence of healing after 6 days of treatment with an antifungal agent
- Presence of more than 2 episodes of vaginitis within 6 months
- Pregnancy
- Sexually transmitted infection suspected
- Patient under 12 years
- Patient with HIV seropositivity, uncontrolled diabetes, or under immunosuppression

References

- Edwards L. The diagnosis and treatment of infectious vaginitis. Dermatol Ther. 2004; 17:102-10.
- Gilbert DN, Moellering RC, Eliopoulos GM, Sande MA. The Sandford guide to antimicrobial therapy; 34th edition. 2004.
- Owen MK, Clenney TL. Management of vaginitis. Am Fam Physician. 2004; 70:2125-32.
- Plourd MD. Practical guide to diagnosis and treating vaginitis. [Internet]. Medscape General Medicine [Updated 1999]. Available from: http://www.medscape.com/viewarticle/408848.
- Sexually transmitted disease treatment guidelines 2002. Morbidity and mortality weekly report, Vol 51-rr6, 10 May 2002.
- Sobel JD. Vaginitis. New Eng J Med. 1997; 337:1896-1903.
- Sobel JD. Vaginitis vulvitis, cervicitis and cutaneous vulval lesions. Dans: Cohen & Powderly. Infectious disease. 2nd edition. St-Louis: Mosby; 2004.

Pediatric Care

Common Cold and Flu
in Children

Overview

Table I: Differences between Adults and Children during a Viral Infection		
Characteristics	**Adults**	**Children < 6 years**
Frequency	2–4 times a year	Once a month from September–April
Fever (> 38°C)	Rare	Frequent the first 3 days
Nasal manifestations	Congestion	Coloured nasal discharge and congestion
Duration	5–7 days	14 days

Table II: Problems Frequently Observed in Pediatrics	
Acute laryngotracheo-bronchitis or croup	• Obstruction of the upper respiratory tract • In children 6 months–3 years because their respiratory tract is narrower • Happens in winter (from October on) • Often preceded by a cold • Coughing fits (hollow, like barking) that start abruptly, often during the night after the child has been sleeping for a few hours • Loss of appetite, general malaise
Cold	• Rhinorrhea and/or nasal congestion, irritated or sore throat • Sneezing • Cough • Fever
Allergies	• Dark lines under the eyes • Frequent headaches without fever • Eyes are often red and swollen; they itch and tear • Constant need to clear throat • Throat is always red

Questions to ask

- ✓ How old is the child? Child's weight?
- ✓ How long has the child had symptoms? When do they occur (e.g., especially at night)?
- ✓ Does the child have any specific medical conditions (e.g., asthma, allergies, diabetes, etc.)?
- ✓ What have you used until now?
- ✓ Does the child go to daycare?
- ✓ Was the child in contact with other infected people?

What to do

Prevention

- Wash toys when they have been handled by more than one person
- Make sure the child eats balanced meals and gets enough rest (14 hours for infants, 11–12 hours for young children, and 8–10 hours for school-age children)
- Throw out used tissue paper and wash hands often
- Use a new toothbrush after a cold or the flu
- Keep the child's vaccinations up to date

Treatment

- Use a cold-air humidifier in the child's room (without adding essential oils or other oil products). For a quick solution, using the shower, fill the bathroom with vapour and let the child breathe the moist air
- Make sure the child drinks plenty of fluids
- Use throat lozenges or ice cubes to soothe a sore throat in children over 4

<u>What to use</u>

- There are many OTC products for the relief of flu and cold symptoms. However, there is little scientific evidence supporting their use in young children

- Nonpharmacological measures are the preferred treatment, and pharmaceutical products should be used only as a last resort or if the child is very distressed by the symptoms (e.g., during the night)

- Chewable tablets often contain aspartame. Aspartame is metabolized to L-phenylalanine and must be avoided in children with phenylketonuria

Table III: Pharmacological Treatments

Agent	Dosage	Comments
	Cough	
Dextromethorphan	1–3 months: 0.5–1 mg q6–8h 3–6 months: 1–2 mg q6–8h 7 months–1 year: 2–4 mg q6–8h ≥ 2–6 years: 2.5–7.5 mg q6–8h or extended release formula 15 mg q12h (max.: 30 mg/24h) 7–12 years: 5–10 mg q4h or 15 mg q6–8h (max.: 60 mg/24 h) > 12 years: 10–30 mg q4–8h or extended release formula 60 mg q12h (max.: 120 mg/24 h)	• The dosage for children < 2 years is not well established, but literature mentions possible use starting at 1 month of age • The American Academy of Pediatrics does not recommend its use in children • Side effects: nausea, dizziness, drowsiness
Codeine	1–1.5 mg/kg/day q4–6h prn OR 2–5 years: 2.5–5 mg q4–6h prn (max.: 30 mg/day) 6–12 years: 5–10 mg q4–6h prn (max.: 60 mg/day) > 12 years: 10–20 mg q4–6h prn (max.: 120 mg/day)	• Not recommended for children under 2 • For dry cough only • Side effects: nausea, vomiting, constipation, pruritus
Guaifenesin	< 2 years: 12 mg/kg/day divided into 6 doses prn (max.: 300 mg/day) 2–5 years: 50–100 mg q4h prn (max.: 600 mg/day) 6–12 years: 100–200 mg q4h prn (max.: 1.2 g/day) > 12 years: 200–400 mg q4h prn (max.: 2.4 g/day)	• Expectorant for productive cough • Combine with plenty of fluids to increase efficacy • Side effects: nausea, drowsiness, headache, dizziness

Table III: Pharmacological Treatments (cont'd)

Agent	Dosage	Comments
Nasal Congestion		
Saline solution 0.9%	1–2 drops or using a vaporizer, spray into each nostril prn (at least 4 times a day or when the child cannot breathe). Leave for a few minutes to soften secretions then remove with a nasal aspirator	• First choice for infants, because they cannot breathe through the mouth and nurse at the same time. The nasal passages must therefore be cleared so infants can breathe while they eat • For infants, use drops because they are less irritating than a vaporizer • Home remedy: ½ tsp. salt in 240 mL water • Side effects: irritation
Pseudoephedrine	< 2 years: 4 mg/kg/day divided q6h prn 2–5 years: 15 mg q6h prn (max.: 60 mg/day) 6–12 years: 30 mg q6h prn (max.: 120 mg/day) > 12 years: 60 mg q6h prn (max.: 240 mg/day)	• Side effects: tachycardia, palpitations, anxiety, nausea, vomiting, insomnia (excitability)
Xylometazoline Topical	2–12 years: 2–3 drops q8h prn pediatric drops 0.05% < 6 years: 1 spray/nostril q8h prn nasal spray 0.05% 6–12 years: 1–2 spray/nostril q6h prn nasal spray 0.05%	• < 6 months: not recommended
Rhinorrhea		
Chlorpheniramine	< 12 years: 0.35 mg/kg/day divided q4–6h **OR** 2–5 years: 1 mg q4–6h 6–11 years: 2 mg q4–6h (max.: 12 mg/day) ≥ 12 years: 4 mg q4–6h (max.: 24 mg/day)	• Side effects: drowsiness, excitability, nausea, diarrhea
Brompheniramine	< 6 years: 0.125 mg/kg q6h (max.: 6–8 mg/day) 6–12 years: 2–4 mg q6–8h (max.: 12–16 mg/day)	• Should not be used in newborns

Table III: Pharmacological Treatments (cont'd)

Agent	Dosage	Comments
Fever and headache		
Acetaminophen	10–15 mg/kg/dose q4–6h (max.: 5 doses/day) Can be used starting at birth	• Side effects: Rash, liver toxicity at high single and cumulative doses
Ibuprofen	5–10 mg/kg/dose q6–8h	• Side effects: dyspepsia, nausea, tinnitus
Allergies		
Diphenhydramine	5 mg/kg/day divided q6–8h (maximum dose: 50 mg. max.: 300 mg/day) OR 2 – < 6 years: 6.25 mg q4–6h (max.: 37.5 mg/day) > 6 years – < 12 years: 12.5 mg q4–6h (max.: 150 mg/day) ≥ 12 years: 25–50 mg q4–6h (max.: 300 mg/day)	• Side effects: drowsiness, irritability, excitability, nausea, diarrhea
Loratadine	2–5 years: 5 mg qd ≥ 6 years: 10 mg qd	• Side effects: dry mouth, fatigue, headache, drowsiness
Desloratadine	6–11 months: 1 mg qd 1–5 years: 1.25 mg po qd 6–11 years: 2.5 mg po qd ≥ 12 years: 5 mg po qd	• Side effects: dry mouth, fatigue, headache, drowsiness
Fexofenadine	6–11 years: 30 mg po bid ≥ 12 years: 60 mg po bid or 180 mg po qd	• Fruit juice can reduce bioavailability by 36% • Side effects: dry mouth, fatigue, headache, drowsiness

When to consult

- Presence of respiratory difficulty (stridor, flaring nostrils)
- Not able to feed the child
- Rhinorrhea for more than 10 days
- Fever for more than 48–72 hours
- Child is a known asthmatic
- If sinus infection or otitis suspected

References

- Dosing of OTC products in the pediatric population. Pharmacist's Letter/Prescriber's Letter 2006; 22:220117.
- Pappas DE, Hendly JO. The common cold. In: Long SS. Principles and practice of pediatric infectious disease. 2nd edition. Philadelphia: PA. Elsevier Science; 2003.
- Roy H. Les médicaments en vente libre réservés à l'usage pédiatrique (Part I), Québec Pharmacie. 2003; 450.
- Roy H. Les médicaments en vente libre réservés à l'usage pédiatrique (Part 2), Québec Pharmacie. 2003; 50.
- Taketomo CK, Hodding JH, Kraus DM. Pediatric dosage handbook 2007, 13th edition.
- Tristram DA, Welliver RC. Bronchiolitis. In: Long SS. Principles and practice of pediatric infectious disease. 2nd edition. Philadelphia: PA. Elsevier Science; 2003.
- Children's relief: Cold and flu. [Internet]. Canada. McNeil Consumer Healthcare. [update 2005 December 1, cited 200 May 21]. Available from: http://www.tylenol.ca/english/faq_list.asp?cfa=4#x4.
- Product monographs. [Internet]. Canada. Rougier Inc. [cited 2007 May 21]. Available from: http://www.balminil.com.

Constipation
in Children

Overview

- Constipation is characterized by the following symptoms:
  - Painful defecation (dyschesia)
  - Frequency of bowel movements < 3 times/week
  - Hard stools

Table I: Normal Frequency of Defecation in Children		
Age	Average number of bowel movements per week	Average number of bowel movements per day
0–3 months: breastfed	5–40	2.9
0–3 months: formula fed	5–28	2.0
6–12 months	5–28	1.8
1–3 years	4–21	1.4
> 3 years	3–14	1.0 .

Adapted from Baker et al.

Questions to ask

✓ **Describe the symptoms**
  - Frequency? Characteristics? Duration?

✓ **What are the possible etiologies?**
  - Constipating medications? Nutrition? Changes in eating habits? Fear of defecating?

✓ **Other associated symptoms?**
  - Abdominal pain? Nocturnal and/or daytime enuresis? Urinary urgency? Mood swings? Aggressiveness?

What to do

- Determine if the problem is organic or functional in nature:
  - <u>Organic causes: rare, but must be excluded as a priority</u>

    For example: anatomic, endocrine, neuromuscular, metabolic causes; lesion of the CNS
  - <u>Functional causes: very frequent (95% of cases) can be related to</u>
    - **a food problem:** introduction of cow's milk, insufficient intake, undernourishment, diet too rich in carbohydrates or in protein (or both), poor in fibre; or
    - **the child's behaviour in facing the pain of passing stools**

What to use

- Nonpharmacological advice must always be given with pharmacological treatment
- If possible, stop administration of any medication likely to cause constipation
- The oral route of administration is the treatment of choice so as to minimize trauma to the anal region and to promote treatment compliance

Table II: Advice to Parents on Nonpharmacological Measures
· Explain the physiopathological characteristics of constipation to the family. Make a drawing of the digestive tract and explain the constipation mechanism and how stools are formed
· Interventions will depend on the age of the child and on the severity of the constipation
· **Newborn**: add brown sugar to formula or to water (1 tsp. in 4–8 oz or 5 mL in 125–250 mL)
· **Infant**: when solid food is added to the diet, gradually increase the proportion of fruits and vegetables to the regimen
· **Child**: prune juice or prunes are sometimes effective
· Stress the importance of a diet rich in fibre, of abundant fluid intake, and increased physical activity
· Teach good toilet-training habits in very young children: regular attempts after meals, good position (hips tilted, feet flat on the ground)
· Stress the importance of positive reinforcement

Table III: Pharmacological Treatments for Constipation in Children

Drugs	Dosage	Side Effects	Comments
Lubricants/Emollients: Soften stool and facilitate evacuation Onset of action: 12–72 hours			

Docusate sodium
(emollient)
	5 mg/kg/day qd-qid	• Mild abdominal cramps
		• Rash
			• First line of treatment
			• Can be administered with milk or fruit juice
			    Colace: 4 mg/mL
			    Colace drops: 10 mg/mL

Mineral oil
(lubricant)
	≤ 1 year: not recommended
	≤5 years: 5 mL po qd
	5–11 years: 5–15 mL/day
	≥12 years: 15–45 mL/day
		• Lipoid pneumonia possible if aspiration
		• In theory, interferes with the absorption of liposoluble vitamins
			• Better tasting if taken cold
			• Avoid in infants
			    Lansoyl (78% mineral oil)
			    Nujol (100% mineral oil)
			    Fleet enema mineral oil (100% mineral oil)

Mucilage: Forms of fibre that, due to their ability to hold water, help increase stool volume and weight associated with shortened stool transit time and more frequent bowel movements Onset of action: 12–24 hours. Peak action: 2–3 days			
Psyllium	<6 years: not recommended 6–11 years: 0.5–1 tsp. in 120 mL of liquid po qd-tid ≥12 years: adult dose	• Abdominal pain	• Safe and effective in children if they take enough, but frequent problem with treatment compliance • Contraindicated if fecal impaction

		Table III: Pharmacological Treatments for Constipation in Children (cont'd)		
Drugs	Dosage	Side Effects	Comments	
Osmotics: Retain fluids in the intestine by osmosis, and change water distribution in stools Onset of action: 1–2 days				
Lactulose	5–10 mL/day qd–qid Double daily until a bowel movement is obtained or 1–3 mL/kg/day in divided doses Max.: 60 mL/day tid–qid	• Bloating • Flatulence • Abdominal cramps	• First line of treatment • *Laxilose* syrup: 65% lactulose • *Lactulose* syrup: 66.7%	
Magnesium citrate	≤ 6 years: 2–4 mL/kg/dose in a single dose or in divided doses Max.: 150 mL 6–12 years: 100–150 mL/dose in a single dose or in divided doses ≥ 12 years: 150–300 mL/day Max.: 300 mL	• Warning: children are more prone to magnesium poisoning (altered mental state, respiratory distress, hypotension)	• Better tasting if taken cold • *Mag-Citrate*: 59 mg/mL	

		Table III: Pharmacological Treatments for Constipation in Children (cont'd)	
Drugs	Dosage	Side Effects	Comments
Magnesium hydroxide	**Dosage based on concentration of milk of magnesia: 80 mg/mL** ≤2 years: 0.5 mL/kg/dose 2–5 years: 5–15 mL/day 6–11 years: 15–30 mL/day ≥12 years: 30–60 mL/day **Dosage based on combination of milk of magnesia and mineral oil:** ≤2 years: 0.6 mL/kg/dose 2–5 years: 5–15 mL/day 6–11 years: 15–30 mL/day ≥12 years: 30–60 mL/day	• Warning: children are more prone to magnesium poisoning (altered mental state, respiratory distress, hypotension)	• Milk of magnesia, liquid: 80 mg/mL *Magnolax*: 300 mg magnesium hydroxide +1.25 mL mineral oil/5 mL • Can decrease absorption of tetracycline, digoxin, isoniazid, quinolones, and iron
Polyethylene glycol (PEG 3350)	Powder to be mixed with water or juice: 0.8–1 g/kg/day in 2 doses. Max. dose: 17 g/day Enema dose: 1–1.5 g/kg/day x 3 days	• Nausea, cramps, abdominal distension, vomiting	• Titrate the dose every 3 days • 17 g is equivalent to approximately one rounded tablespoon • Solution can be prepared 1–2 days in advance • Certain data suggest that PEG is more effective than Lactulose • Recommended for chronic constipation

Table III: Pharmacological Treatments for Constipation in Children (cont'd)

Drugs	Dosage	Side Effects	Comments
Fleet (Na phosphate)	≤ 2 years: not recommended **Oral:** 5–9 years: 5 mL po in a single dose 10–12 years: 10 mL po in a single dose **Intrarectal:** 2–11 years: *Fleet* pediatric (60 mL) PR prn ≥ 12 years: *Fleet* adult (135 mL) PR prn	• Abdominal distension • Hyperphosphatemia, hypokalemia, and hypocalcemia if retention • Risk of mechanical trauma	• Precaution if renal dysfunction and Hirschsprung's disease • *Fleet* oil form: emollient for hardened stools • *Fleet* phosphate: stimulant of rectal peristalsis
Stimulants: Stimulate production of fluids in the intestine as well as nerve endings in the intestinal wall, which promotes peristalsis. Onset of action: 6–12 hours **Use for a short period only (< 1 week). Not recommended in cases of chronic constipation**			
Sennosides	1 month–2 years: 2.125–8.6 mg po qd Max. dose: 8.6 mg 2–6 years: 4.3 mg–8.6 mg qd Max. dose: 17.2 mg 6–12 years: 8.6 mg–17.2 mg qd Max. dose: 34 mg	• Discolouration of urine and feces • Abdominal cramps • Nausea/vomiting • Hypokalemia	• *Senokot* syrup: 8.6 mg/5 mL • Senna tablets: 8.6 mg/tablet, sennosides

Table III: Pharmacological Treatments for Constipation in Children (cont'd)

Drugs	Dosage	Side Effects	Comments
Bisacodyl	**Oral:** 0.3 mg/kg/day qd or 3–12 years: 5–10 mg ≥12 years: 5–15 mg/day Max. dose: 30 mg **Intrarectal:** <2 years: 5 mg/day 2–11 years: 5–10 mg/day	• Abdominal cramps • Nausea/vomiting • Hypokalemia	• Bisacodyl suspension: 2 mg/mL • Bisacodyl tablets: 5 or 10 mg/tablet • Bisacodyl suppositories: 10 mg • *Dulcolax* micro-enema
Other			
Glycerin suppositories	<6 years: 1 pediatric suppository, prn >6 years: 1 adult suppository, prn	• Local irritation	• Useful during dyschesia • Suppository for child: 1.44 g • Suppository for adult: 2.6 g

When to consult

- Complicated functional constipation suspected: presence of fecal impaction and encopresis (regular expulsion of formed or semi-formed stools in underwear by a child 4 years or older)

- Organic cause suspected

- The following signs and symptoms: vomiting, abdominal pain, delayed evacuation of meconium at birth, fever, pain, bloating, bloody diarrhea, constipation since birth, abdominal tenderness, mass or distended abdomen, fatigue, delayed growth, weight loss

- Failure of treatments

References

- Baker S, Liptak G, Colletti R, Croffie J, Dilorenzo C., Ector W, et al. Constipation in infants and children: Evaluation and treatment. A medical position statement of the North American Society for Pediatric Gastroenterology and Nutrition. Algorithm for Evaluation and Treatment for Constipation.
- Biggs W, Dery W. Evaluation and treatment of constipation in infants and children. American Academy of Family Physicians 2006; 73: 469-77.
- Bell E. Pediatric Constipation therapy using guidelines and polyethylene glycol 3350. The Annals of Pharmacotherapy. 2004; 38:686-693.
- Clinical Practice Guideline. Evaluation and treatment of constipation in infants and children: recommendations of the North American Society for Pediatric Gastroenterology, Hepatology and Nutrition. Journal of Pediatric Gastroenterology and Nutrition. 2006; 43: e1-e13.
- Felt B, Wise C, Olson A, et al. Guidelines for the management of pediatric idiopathic constipation and soiling. Archives Pediatric Adolescent 1999; 153;380-385.
- Felt B, Brown P, et al. Functional constipation and soiling in children. Clinics in family and practice 2004; 6:709-30.
- Rubin G, Dale A. Chronic constipation in children. BMJ. 2006; 333:1051-1055.
- Taketomo C, Hodding J, Kraus D. Pediatric dosage handbook 13th edition. Lexi-Comp Drug Information Series; 2006-2007.
- Youssef N, Di Lorenzo C. Childhood constipation. Journal Clinical Gastroenterology. 2001; 33:199-205.

Fever and Febrile Seizures
in Children

Overview

Fever

- Body temperature higher than:
  - 38.2°C (rectal)
  - 37.5°C (oral)
  - 37.2°C (axillary)

Table I: Taking a Child's Temperature
· Method of choice based on age:
○ < 2 years: rectal temperature, tympanic temperature (an alternative only);
○ 2–5 years: rectal, tympanic, axillary temperature;
○ > 5 years: oral temperature, except if the child cannot keep its mouth closed long enough. Other possibilities: axillary and tympanic
· Taking axillary temperature is not recommended because there is a risk of underestimating the readings; use oral, rectal, or tympanic measurement
· Avoid using rectal measurement for patients taking chemotherapy
· Regardless of the method chosen, ensure that the parent knows how to take the child's temperature accurately

Table II: Advice for Parent on Taking a Child's Temperature
Rectal measurement
· Lubricate the end of the thermometer with a hydrosoluble lubricating gel
· Place the infant on your knees, supporting its head, or lay it flat on its stomach on a flat, hard surface
· Immobilize the infant by placing the palm of your hand on its lower back
· With the other hand, introduce the lubricated thermometer into the infant's rectum, to a depth of about 1.25–2.5 cm. In the event of resistance, stop at 1.25 cm
· Hold the thermometer in place with your fingers while supporting your hand on the infant's buttocks
Tympanic measurement
· According to manufacturer's instructions. The probe must be correctly positioned in the ear canal
Axillary measurement
· Remove clothing from the child's torso. The thermometer must be in contact only with skin, not clothing
· Place the thermometer in the child's armpit
· Press the child's arm against its torso so as to keep the thermometer in place
Oral measurement
· Ensure that the child's mouth is free of candy, gum, or food
· Place the end of the thermometer under the child's tongue and make sure the child keeps it in place with the lips
· Remind the child not to bite the thermometer and not to talk while temperature is being taken

Causes

- Infections
- Drug fever
- Central nervous system (CNS) etiology

Questions to ask

✓ **How long has the child presented with fever?**

✓ **What are the temperature readings?**

✓ **What are the other symptoms?**

✓ **What is the child's drug history?**

What to do

Table III: Nonpharmacological Measures
• Give the child plenty of fluids to prevent dehydration and to help control body temperature
• Have the child rest; moving can increase body temperature
• Keep room temperature between 21 °C and 23 °C
• Dress the child lightly (e.g., light cotton pyjamas) to allow body heat to escape
• If the child is shivering, add a blanket; and remove it when shivering stops
• It is useless to give the child a warm bath or to sponge the child. This can cause shivering and increase rather than decrease temperature
• Do not use rubbing alcohol to bring temperature down

What to use

• Acetaminophen and ibuprofen: comparable efficacy and safety

• Use dosage by weight. The dosage on the package (by age) may underestimate or overestimate the dose

• Avoid ASA for children under 18 because of the risk of Reye's syndrome

Table IV: Treating Fever		
Agents	**Dosage**	**Comments**
Acetaminophen *(Tylenol)*	**< 1 month:** 10–15 mg/kg q6h prn (max. 65 mg/kg/day) **> 1 month–12 years:** 10–15 mg/kg q4–6h (max. 75 mg/kg/day or 5 doses/day) **> 12 years** (adult doses): 325–650 mg q4–6h prn Max. 4 g/day	• Very well tolerated in children • Avoid overdoses because there is a risk of liver toxicity
Ibuprofen *(Motrin, Advil)*	5–10 mg/kg q6–8h (max. 4 doses/day)	• Not indicated as an OTC product for children under 2 • Very well tolerated in children

When to consult

- Under 2 years
- Fever over 40.5° C
- Very sick/inconsolable child
- Stiff neck, seizures, redness, edema
- Confusion
- Patient taking chemotherapy
- Fever persisting for more than 24 hours
- Fever unresolved after 72 hours

Febrile Seizures

Overview

- Definition: seizures associated with fever in the absence of evidence of infection of the CNS (encephalitis, meningitis) or other causes (neurological trauma, encephalopathy) in a child aged 1 month to 5 years without a history of nonfebrile epileptic seizure

- Distinguish between two possible scenarios:

  1) Febrile seizures: transitory, benign manifestations occurring during a quick, pronounced rise in temperature

  2) Epilepsy: first seizures can evoke febrile seizures because their first manifestation occurs during an episode of fever

- Incidence: 2–5% in children 6 months to 5 years of age. The age of onset is usually between 6 months and 3 years, with a peak at 18 months

- Recurrence: One third of children will develop a second episode

- Antipyretics must be used to treat fever; they are not effective in preventing the recurrence of febrile seizures

- Risk factors

  o Viral infections

  o Vaccination: tetanus (D_2T_5), MMR. Febrile seizures occur within 48 hours following vaccination

  o Family history (first degree) of febrile seizures or epilepsy

What to do

- All cases of febrile seizures must be referred to a physician to clarify the type (simple or complex febrile seizures) and to exclude any other diagnosis

- Reassure the parents because most febrile seizures are without sequella for the child

Table V: Advice to Parents Regarding Febrile Seizures
· Febrile seizures are a common phenomenon and usually benign; the risk of damage to the brain and of epilepsy is very rare. The mortality rate is virtually nil
· Febrile seizures can manifest as follows: body rigidity, rolling eyes, disorderly movement of limbs, loss of consciousness
· The seizures generally last 1 minute but can last up to 15 minutes. If the seizures last more than 5 minutes, call an ambulance
· Apply the usually necessary measures during the seizures: place the child in a safe lateral position on the ground to avoid a fall; remove dangerous objects; do not put anything in the child's mouth
· Because fever is the trigger for seizures, it is important to limit the fever using antipyretics. Their efficacy is however not known in the prevention of recurrence of febrile seizures
· Genetic transmission is unknown, but 25–40% of children affected have a positive family history

References

- Carmant L. Les convulsions fébriles chez l'enfant. Le clinicien 2002; March: 81-9.
- El-Radhi AS, Barry W. Thermometry in paediatric practice. Arch Dis Child. 2006; 91: 351-6.
- Langley JM. Fever in children. n: Gray J, editor. Therapeutic choices. 3rd edition. Ottawa: Canadian Pharmacists Association; 2000. p. 882-4.
- Pearce C, Curtis N. Fever in children. Australian Family Physician. 2005; 34:769-71.
- Rosman P. Evaluation of the child who convulses with fever. Pediatric Drugs. 2003; 5:457-61.
- Shevchuk Y. Fever. In: Repchinsky C, Leblanc C, editors. Patient self-care: helping patients make therapeutic choices. 1st edition. Ottawa: Canadian Pharmacists Association; Welcom Ltd: 2002. p. 79-90.
- Srinivasan J, Wallace K, Scheffer I. Febrile seizures. Aust Fam Physician. 2005; 34:1021-25.
- Warden CR, Zibulewsky J, Sharon M, Gold C, Marianne GH. Evaluation and management of febrile seizures in the out-of-hospital and emergency department settings. Ann Emerg Med. 2003 ;41: 512-22.
- Waruiru C, Appleton R. Febrile seizures: an update. Arch Dis Child. 2004; 89:751-6.

Gastroenteritis
in Children

Overview

- Inflammation (usually infectious) of the digestive tract resulting in diarrhea and vomiting

- Condition is very frequent, especially among infants

- The risk of dehydration attributable to diarrhea is much higher in children than in adults, given the difference in body water content and body weight/surface ratio

Questions to ask

✓ **What are the symptoms? (diarrhea, vomiting, weight loss, mood changes, lethargy, apathy, etc.)**

✓ **Specify the frequency, volume, and duration of vomiting and diarrhea to determine the severity of fluid depletion and electrolytic imbalance**

✓ **Changes in diet?**

✓ **History of illness in those close to the child, including playmates, brothers and sisters, and daycare employees?**

✓ **Recent use of antibiotics?**

What to do

- **Before concluding gastroenteritis, ensure that diarrhea is not being caused by the child's diet. If diet is the cause:**

  o Limit the consumption of juice or sweet fluids: limit to 60–90 mL per day until the child is 2 years old

  o Avoid skim milk and food that is too cold

  o Temporarily stop giving any new foods

- o In accordance with age and tolerance, add a little fat (margarine, butter) to food, because it slows intestinal transit time

- o If diarrhea is light, it is not necessary to change the child's diet

- **Evaluate dehydration and choose an oral rehydration solution (ORS)**

  - o Begin oral rehydration promptly

- **Avoid spreading**

  - o In order to avoid spreading gastroenteritis, encourage frequent hand washing

What to use

| | | | | | | | | Table I: Evaluation and Treatment of Dehydration | | | |
Dehydration (% loss)	General State	Thirst	Eyes and Tearing	Mouth	Skin	Urine	Rehydration within 4 hours?	Replacement of Hydric Losses
None (< 2%)	Well, alert	Drinks Normally	Normal, presence of tears	Moist	Normal	Normal	Not necessary; begin with maintenance treatment to replace current losses	10 mL/hr or ½ to 1 cup of ORS for each diarrhea bowel movement; from 2–5 mL/kg for each vomiting episode
Mild (3–5%)	Well	Drinks eagerly	Normal, fewer tears	Less moist	Normal	Decreased	ORS, 50 mL/kg	As above
Moderate (6–9%)	Restless, irritable	Drinks eagerly	Sunken, dry	Dry	Pale, vascular filling* and skin fold recall tests: < 2 seconds**	Absent	ORS, 100 mL/kg	As above
Serious (>= 10%)	Lethargy, diminished awareness, rapid weak pulse, shallow breathing	Drinks little or is unable to drink	Very sunken and dry, no tears	Very dry	Pale, vascular filling* and skin fold recall tests: > 2 seconds**	Absent	IV fluids Take to the hospital	As above

ORS: Oral rehydration solution

* briefly press on child's nail bed so that it blanches or turns white, and see how long it takes to return to normal

** gently pinch child's skin on their abdomen, hold it for a few seconds and then let go to see how long it takes to return to the normal position

Table II: Composition of Oral Rehydration Solutions and Drinks						
Solution	Carbo-hydrates (g/L)	Sodium (mmol/L)	Potassium (mmol/L)	Chloride (mmol/L)	Base (mmol/L)	Osmo-larity (mOsm/L)
WHO (2002 formula)	13.5	75	20	65	30	245
Enfalyte	30	50	25	45	34	200
Gastrolyte	17.8	60	20	60	10	240
Pedialyte	25	45	20	35	30	250
Solutions not recommended as alternatives for ORS						
Apple juice	120	0.4	44	45	n/a	730
Coca-Cola	112	1.6	n/a	n/a	13.4	650

Adapted from Butzner (2006)

Oral rehydration solutions

- Commercial preparations: do not add juice to improve the taste

- Home remedy: 360 mL unsweetened orange juice without pulp + 600 mL boiled water + 2.5 mL salt

- To reduce the risk of error, it is preferable to use a ready-to-use solution rather than one requiring dilution. Administration of a rehydration solution is effective even if the child vomits, unless there is uncontrolled vomiting

- Avoid apple juice, carbonated drinks, and sports drinks such as Gatorade. They can aggravate the electrolytic and mineral imbalance (inadequate quantities of sugar and sodium)

- Antidiarrhea and antiemetic agents are not recommended

Encourage prompt food replenishment

- Foods to avoid are those rich in simple sugars, drinks containing caffeine, presweetened gelatins and sugar-coated cereals

- Foods rich in fats may not be well tolerated because of the delay in gastric emptying that provokes increased vomiting

- Do not give tap water to children with acute gastroenteritis so as to avoid hyponatremia and hypoglycemia

Children of all ages

- If breastfeeding, continue with breastfeeding. Between feedings, give a rehydration solution by spoon or by dropper (5–10 mL) every 5–10 minutes

- If bottle fed, stop usual feeding (milk and solids) for approximately 4 hours. Between feedings, give a rehydration solution by spoon or by dropper (5–10 mL) every 5–10 minutes

- These measures (liquid diet without milk or solid food) generally last 6–12 hours and must not be maintained for more than 18 hours

- Monitor closely for signs and symptoms of dehydration described below. In the presence of these signs or symptoms, consult a physician

- Adding a new food is not recommended

When to consult

- Signs of dehydration: drowsiness, lethargy, apathy, depression of fontanel in young infants (up to 6 months), dryness of the mouth, circles under the eyes, less frequent micturation and darker urine, absence of tears when crying

- High fever (> 38°C children < 3 months, > 39°C children 3–36 months

- Young infants (< 6 months)

- Significant vomiting or diarrhea

- Signs of mental alteration, blood in stools or in vomit

- Gastric malaise and persistent diarrhea despite taking measures mentioned above

References

- Butzner, J.D. Acute vomiting and diarrhea. In: Walker-Smith JA, Walker WA, Hamilton JR, editors. Practical pediatric gastroenterology, 2nd edition. Toronto: BC Decker; 1996. p. 51-69.
- Butzner J.D, Acute Diarrhea in Children. [Internet]. In: Thomson ABR. Shaffer EA, editors. First Principles of Gastroenterology: The Basis of Disease and an Approach to Management. Chapter 15; 593-. [cited 2007 May 13]. Available at: http://www.gastroresource.com/GITextbook/en/Chapter15/15-6.htm.
- King CK, Glass R, Bresee JS, Duggan C. Managing acute gastroenteritis among children oral rehydration, maintenance, and nutritional therapy. MMWR Recomm Rep. 2003; 52:1-16.
- Elliott EJ. Acute gastroenteritis in children. BMJ. 2007 Jan 6; 334: 35-40.
- Sandhu BK. European Society of Paediatric Gastroenterology, Hepatology, and Nutrition Working Group on Acute Diarrhoea. Rationale for early feeding in childhood gastroenteritis. J Pediatr Gastroenterol Nutr. 2001; 33:S13-6.
- Sandhu BK. Practical guidelines for the management of gastroenteritis in children. J Pediatr Gastroenterol Nutr. 2001; 33: S36-9.
- Canadian Paediatric Society. Oral rehydration therapy and early refeeding in the management of childhood gastroenteritis. Paediatrics & Child Health. 2006; 11 (8): 527-531.
- Szajewska H, Hoekstra JH, Sandhu B. Management of acute gastroenteritis in Europe and the impact of the new recommendations: a multicenter study. The Working Group on acute Diarrhoea of the European Society for Paediatric Gastroenterology, Hepatology, and Nutrition. J Pediatr Gastroenterol Nutr 2000; 30: 522-7.

Infant Formulas
and Nutrition

Overview

Breastfeeding

- Breastfeeding exclusively for the first 6 months should always be encouraged before giving any advice on infant formula, except in cases of contraindication

- Starting at the age of 6 months, the introduction of solid foods high in nutritional value, especially iron, is recommended, while continuing to breastfeed until the age of 2 years and even beyond

- Breastfed infants should also be given daily Vitamin D supplements until their food contains adequate amounts, or until age 1. It is recommended that all healthy breastfed full-term newborns receive a supplement of 10 µg/day (400 IU/day) of Vitamin D. For children over 1, the daily Vitamin D supplement should be 5 µg (200 IU)

Breastfeeding contraindications

- The mother has HIV/AIDS
- The mother is undergoing chemotherapy or taking cytotoxic medication
- The mother has breast cancer
- The mother is taking contraindicated drugs
- The infant has galactosemia (problem metabolizing galactose)

Medications that are Contraindicated or to be used with Precaution when Breastfeeding

- Some anticonvulsants
- Antineoplastics

- Illicit drugs

- Ergot alkaloids (at dosages for treating migraines)

- Medications causing lactation suppression (e.g., cabergoline, bromocriptine)

- Radioactive compounds (e.g., strontium-89, thallium-201) (temporarily interrupt breastfeeding)

- Amiodarone (monitor the infant's serum levels and thyroid function)

- Cyclosporine (monitor the mother and infant's serum levels and signs of immunosuppression, especially, infections and an abnormal CBC

- Azathioprine (monitor the mother's serum levels and signs of immunosuppression in the infant)

- Lithium (monitor the mother and infant's serum levels and ensure the infant receives adequate fluids)

- Oral contraceptives containing estrogen (ensure that the quantity of milk is sufficient; monitor the infant's weight gain)

Alcohol and Breastfeeding

- Regular consumption exceeding 0.5 g/kg/day, about two drinks, is contraindicated

- According to the Motherisk Program (The Hospital for Sick Children, Toronto), nursing should be withheld temporarily, two hours for every drink taken

Advice to Mothers in cases of Nursing Strike

- Temporary events that may have many causes: mother's menstruation, change in the mother's diet, use of a new soap, teething, or illness

- Possible measures to take

  o Make breastfeeding time special and quiet and reduce distractions to a minimum

  o Increase the amount of cuddling and soothing of the baby

- o Offer the breast when the infant is very sleepy or when just waking up
- o Do not attempt to "starve" the infant into submission
- o Offer the breast frequently using different nursing positions, alternating sides. Try nursing in different rooms
- If the above steps do not result in re-establishing of breastfeeding, then the infant should be evaluated to rule out possible illness

Infant Formulas

- Commercial formulas are the best replacement milk until the age of 9–12 months for infants who are breastfed in part, or not breastfed

General recommendations

- Use iron-fortified, cow-milk based infant formula until the age of 9–12 months
- Choose transition formulas fortified with iron rather than cow's milk for infants from the age of 6–9 months
- Pasteurized whole cow's milk (3.25%) can be given to infants from the age of 9 months on (partially skimmed and skimmed milk are not recommended during the first 2 years of life)
- Unpasteurized cow's and goat's milk is contraindicated
- Use soy-based formulas only for infants who cannot consume milk products for reasons related to health, culture or religion, like the practice of veganism or the presence of galactosemia
- Use special formulas for infants with a diagnosed or presumed pathology
- Soy beverages (with the exception of soy-based formulas), rice beverages, or other vegetarian beverages, enriched or not, are not appropriate substitutes
- Home-made formulas made from condensed milk (cow or goat) are not recommended as substitutes

Recommendations Regarding Other Liquids for Feeding Infants

- Boil at a rolling boil for at least 2 minutes any water used for feeding infants under 4 months so as to eliminate all pathogenic agents

- Limit fruit juices to avoid adversely affecting the ingestion of breast milk or of infant formula

- Do not give infants herbal teas or other beverages

What to do

- Wash the top of the can of formula before opening it

- Always provide advice on the instructions of the infant formula chosen: if the solution is too concentrated, there will be a risk of dehydration; and if it is too diluted, there will be a risk of malnutrition

- Water for preparing formula for infants <u>under 4 months</u> must be sterilized

  o Tap, well, or bottled water must be boiled for 5 minutes. This water can be kept for 48–72 hours in the refrigerator in a sterile container or for 24 hours at room temperature

- The milk must always be at room temperature

  o To warm formula, fill the bottle and soak in hot tap water for a few minutes. Never use the microwave oven to avoid the risk of burns

- Once formula has been prepared, it can keep for 24–48 hours in the fridge or for approximately 1 hour at room temperature

- Do not freeze

What to use

- The choice depends mainly on the infant's health, the risk of allergies, and the cost

Table I: Infant Formulas

Composition	Brand Name	Characteristics
Cow's milk with protein and lactose	*Enfalac* *Enfalac with Iron* *Enfamil A+ (enriched with DHA and ARA)* *Nestlé Good Start* *Similac Advance* *Similac Advance With Iron* *SMA regular* *SMA fortified with iron*	• **1st choice**, except if the infant has galactosemia or presents with a diagnosed allergy to cow milk protein • Non-iron-enriched formulas are preferable for infants exclusively breastfed who take formula from time to time (because breast milk provides enough iron). Otherwise, choose an iron-enriched formula for all children unless contraindicated • DHA and ARA: omega-3 and -6 fatty acids promote development of the eyes and brain
Cow's milk with protein, lactose FREE	*Enfalac Lactofree* *Similac LF*	• Primary lactose intolerance is very rare and should be confirmed by a pediatrician before suggesting a lactose-free formula • The glucose polymers in corn syrup replace lactose • Ideal for children presenting with lactose intolerance • Not for children presenting with galactosemia

Table I: Infant Formulas (cont'd)

Composition	Brand Name	Characteristics
Cow's milk with hydrolized protein	*Enfalac Nutramigen* *Enfalac Pregestimil*	• The protein is predigested • Whey-based: less predigested (controversial for children at risk of allergies) • Casein-based: more predigested (for infants diagnosed as allergic to cow's milk protein or soy milk protein) • Use with caution because some infants can still have an allergic reaction • Can be used for infants with galactosemia
Soy protein	*Enfalac Prosobee soy* *Isomil* *Nestlé Alsoy*	• Lactose free • For infants on a vegetarian diet or with galactosemia • Use is controversial for infants who are allergic to cow's milk protein or for the prevention of allergies • Infants allergic to cow's milk protein can also develop allergies to soy protein
Other formulas	Cow's milk: *Enfalac Next Step* *Nestlé Follow-up* *Similac Advance Step 2* Soy milk: *Nestlé Follow-up Soy*	• **Are not** superior to starter formulas (appropriate formulas until the age of 12 months) • Alternative after age 6 months for infants on solid foods who are not breast fed or who are only breast fed in part
Thickened formulas	*Enfalac AR* (Warning: cow's milk based) *Enfamil Thickened A+*	• Developed for children with gastroesophageal reflux or who regurgitate more than 4 times a day • This advantage can be lost if taking medication that increases gastric pH (H_2-receptor antagonists, PPI)
High-calorie formulas	*Enfalac Enfacare A+*	• For premature babies, or babies with low birth weight, nutrient-enriched • 22 calories per ounce of formula (compared with 20 calories per ounce for other ordinary formulas)

Introduction of Solid Food According to Age

GENERAL RECOMMENDATIONS

- At the age of 6 months, introduce additional foods high in nutrients to meet rising nutritional needs and to promote development
- First, introduce foods rich in iron to avoid iron deficiency
- Introduce one new food at a time, every 3 days, so as to ensure that the infant is not allergic
- Birth–6 months
  - o Breastfeeding or formula only
- 6 months
  - o Give on a teaspoon so that the infant can learn other ways of eating
  - o Breastfeeding or infant formulas PLUS
  - o Iron-fortified semi-liquid rice cereal THEN
  - o Other semi-liquid cereals (oat, barley)
  - o Start with 1 teaspoon of cereal mixed with 4–5 teaspoons of breast milk or formula, once a day, then gradually increase the consistency and the frequency to bid
- 6–8 months
  - o Same as for 6 months
  - o Introduce vegetable purée (well-cooked carrots, squash, avocado, and sweet potato)
  - o Introduce fruit purée (banana, pear, apple compote, peach)
  - o 3–9 teaspoons of cereal per day (divided in bid–tid)
  - o 1 teaspoon of vegetables and 1 teaspoon of fruit (increase gradually)
- 8–10 months
  - o Same as for 6–8 months
  - o Small amounts of milk products (pasteurized mild cheese, low-fat yogurt, cottage cheese)
  - o Wheat cereal and mixed cereal

- o Lightly toasted bagel, small pieces of ripe banana, well-cooked pasta spirals
- o Egg yolk, puréed meat and chicken, pureed potato, tofu, well-cooked peas, mashed
- o Apple or pear juice (no citrus fruits)

- **10–12 months**
  - o Same as for 8–10 months
  - o Fruit cut into cubes or mashed
  - o Bite-sized pieces of cooked vegetables (carrots, peas)
  - o Finely ground meat and/or chicken, lightly toasted bread

- **12–18 months**
  - o Same as for 10–12 months
  - o Whole milk, whole-wheat bread
  - o New fruit: melon, papaya, apricot, grapefruit and other citrus fruits
  - o New vegetables: broccoli, cauliflower
  - o Boned fish
  - o Light spreading of peanut butter
  - o Honey and egg white
  - o Be careful because there is still a risk of choking

- **18–24 months**
  - o Same as for 12–18 months
  - o Hard cheese, yogurt, pudding
  - o Crackers, pretzels, rice, pasta
  - o Cooked, canned, or fresh fruit (strawberries, cherries, grapes, plums, oranges)

Note: This guide makes suggestions. The introduction of some foods may vary according to the reference consulted

References

- American Academy of Pediatrics Section on Breastfeeding. Breastfeeding and the use of human milk. Pediatrics. 2005;115: 496-506.
- Berardi R.R., Mc Dermott J.H., Newton B.D. et al. Handbook of nonprescription drugs: an interactive approach to self-care. 14th edition. APhA. 2004.
- Bernier A. Les préparations lactées. Québec Pharmacie. 2003; 50: 450-4.
- Repchinsky C, Welbanks L, Bisson R, Dang T, Fortin K, Jovaisas B, et al. Compendium of self-care products: the Canadian reference to OTCs. Ottawa: Canadian Pharmacists Association; 2002-3
- Repchinsky C, Leblanc C, editors. Patient self-care: helping patients make therapeutic choices. 1st edition. Ottawa: Canadian Pharmacists Association; Welcom Ltd: 2002. p. 622-46.
- Nutrition for Healthy Term Infants—Statement of the Joint Working Group: Canadian Paediatric Society, Dietitians of Canada, and Health Canada. Minister of Public Works and Government Services Canada, 2005.
- Exclusive Breastfeeding Duration—2004 Health Canada Recommendation. [Internet]. Canada. Health Canada. [cited 2007 May 21]. Available from: http://www.hc-sc.gc.ca/fn-an/nutrition/child-enfant/infant-nourisson/excl_bf_dur-dur_am_excl_e.html.
- Wight N.E. Management of common breastfeeding issues. Pediatr. Clin. North Am. 2001; 48:321-44.
- World Health Organization. Promoting proper feeding for infants and young children. 2003. [Internet]. Geneva. World Health Organization. [cited 2007 May 21]. Available from: http://www.who.int/nutrition/publications/infantfeeding/en/index.html

Infantile Colic

Overview

- **"Rule of three" definition:** Crying that lasts 2–3 hours, 3 times a week, for more than 3 weeks in an infant who is otherwise healthy. The etiology of colic is unknown and often multifactorial

Questions to ask

✓ **What are the symptoms?**

    o Crying and/or irritability for several hours/days, especially in the evening

✓ **Duration of symptoms?**

✓ **Number of hours of crying a day?**

✓ **Crying schedule?**

✓ **Change in feeding method?**

✓ **Methods used to calm the infant?**

What to do

- Relieve parents of their feelings of guilt; reassure them by explaining that they are not the cause of the colic

- Explain the natural history of the infant's colic (frequency and duration) and reassure parents, because the problem usually disappears by itself around age 3–4 months

- In order to have an accurate description of the duration of the crying, ask the mother to keep a journal for a few days

- Colic occurs as frequently among newborns that are breast fed as among newborns that are formula fed

- Try various ways of calming the infant (e.g., carrying in a baby carrier, taking a car ride, or using an automatic cradle or rocker)

- The diet of the breastfeeding mother may influence the presence of colic. Current data on the benefits of a hypoallergenic diet for breastfeeding mothers are inconclusive, but suggest a beneficial effect. The same holds true for hypoallergenic formulas

- Formula of hydrolized casein for the infant or a diet free of milk products for the breastfeeding mother may be useful, especially in the presence of additional symptoms suggesting a food allergy

What to use

- There is no pharmacological treatment of proven efficacy

- Colic generally resolves spontaneously around age 4 months

- Alternative solutions such as herbal tea or Gripe water have not been formally evaluated

Table I: Pharmacological Treatment of Colic			
Drug	Dosage	Side Effects	Comments
Simethicone (Ovol)	< 2 years: 20 mg qid (pc + hs) 2–12 years: 40 mg qid (pc + hs) max.: 240 mg/day	Diarrhea, nausea, vomiting, regurgitation	Current data do not conclusively show the benefits of simethicone in treating colic
Dicyclomine (Bentylol)	6 months–2 years: 5–10 mg tid–qid ac max.: 40 mg/day 2–12 years: 10 mg tid (15 min) ac	Constipation, nausea, drowsiness, apnea, tachycardia	Contraindicated in infants < 6 months because of the risk of apnea Treatment for colic is not an official indication

When to consult

- Vomiting, significant diarrhea
- Increased irritability when the infant is picked up or touched
- Signs and symptoms of mental alteration

References

- Crotteau C, Towner S. What is the best treatment for infants with colics J Fam Pract. Jul 2006; 55: 1-4.
- Ellet ML.C. What is known about infant colic. Gastroenterol Nurs 2003; 26: 60-7.
- Garrison MM, Christakis DA. A systematic review of treatments for infant colic. Pediatrics. 2000; 106:184-90.
- Roberts D, Ostapchuk M, O'Brien J. Infantile colic. American Academy of Family Physician. 2004; 70:735-740.
- Rogovik A. Goldman R. Treating infant's colic. Can Fam Physician 2005; 51:1209-11.

Teething Pain
Teething Pain

Questions to ask

✓ **What are the perceived symptoms? (See Table I)**
✓ **What is the child's age?**
✓ **What measures were used?**

Table I: Symptoms that Can Accompany Teething
· Pain
· Inflammation of the gums
· Malaise/irritability/agitation
· Flushed face/circumoral rash
· Sialorrhea/excessive salivation
· Rubbing the gums
· Gastrointestinal disorders (from constipation to diarrhea)
· Loss of appetite/change in volume of fluids ingested
· Altered sleep
· Rubbing ear on same side as tooth eruption
· Increase in body temperature but seldom > 38.1 °C

What to do

* Teething ring (cold). Avoid rings that contain water because of the risk of bacterial contamination, and rings that can hurt the gums. Choose rings made of solid silicone because they do not leak if pierced and they can be sterilized

* Pacifier

* Cold objects (ice cubes in a plastic hermetically sealed bag or wrapped in soft cloth, cold fruits or vegetables)

* Flush gums with water

* Reassure the parents

What to use

- Teething management consists mainly of relieving the symptoms

- **Analgesics:** Acetaminophen, ibuprofen. For dosages, see the chapter "Pain"

- **Topical anesthetics**: Apply on oral mucosa. No eating for one hour following application. Benzocaine may be more appropriate than lidocaine which can be absorbed significantly by the child. Nevertheless, no benefit has been demonstrated

When to consult

- Significant weight loss

- Significant systemic symptoms

- Prolonged use of a pacifier > 12 months

- Frequent consumption of drinks and snacks

- Visible plaque

References

- A practical guide to infant oral health. American Family Physician. 2004; 70;11:21132120.
- Arthur N, John J. Preventive dental care and counseling for infants and young children. [Internet]. Uptodate. [cited 2007 May 20]. Available from: www.uptodate.com.
- Hass D. An update on analgesics for the management of acute postoperative dental pain. Journal of the Canadian Dental Association. 2002; 68: 476-82.
- McIntyre GT. McIntyre GM. Teething problem? Br. Dent Journal. March 2002; 92: 251-5.

Diagnostic Tests

Ovulation Tests

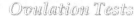

Overview

- The ovulation test works by detecting the lutenizing hormone (LH) in urine

- LH is present throughout the menstrual cycle but its secretion increases abruptly in the 16–36 hours preceding ovulation, that is, just before it

Immunological ovulation test

- This test uses an immunological reaction using monoclonal antibodies

Digital ovulation test

- The _Clear Plan Easy_ fertility monitor indicates the period of fertility by detecting changes in urinary concentrations of estrone-3-glucuronide (metabolite of estradiol), and of LH. It must be used with test strips

- The digital ovulation test is more expensive (about $150 for the device and $1.50/strip)

- Some factors can contribute to incorrect results: taking some medications and the presence of some systemic diseases

Questions to ask

✓ **Is pregnancy wanted?**

   o   Ovulation tests were not designed to serve as a contraceptive method

✓ **Medications taken by the patient?**

- o *Pergonal*, clomiphene, some antiparkinsonians, antipsychotics, and anticonvulsants can increase secretion of LH without necessarily being associated with ovulation

✓ **Presence of systemic diseases?**

- o Renal or hepatic dysfunction can cause the concentration of estrone-3-glucuronide in the urine to vary

- o As well, endometriosis, ovarian cysts, polycystic ovary syndrome, menopause, recent pregnancy, and thyroid disorders can cause a decrease in the concentration of LH in the blood and reduce the reliability of the results

What to do

- Check the expiry date

- Carefully read the manufacturer's instructions. Incorrect use of the test can lead to an incorrect result

- Comply with the required contact time between the urine and the stick or pad as well as the interval before taking a reading because they may vary depending on the test

- If the test chosen requires urine collection, use the cup that comes with the test. Do not clean it with detergent because this could interfere with test results

- Begin the series of daily tests 2–3 days before expected ovulation (see Table I) and follow the manufacturer's instructions to determine this period

- Always do the test at the same time of day

- The ideal time to do the test is 14:00. LH production in women increases in the morning but the increase only appears a few hours later

- Decrease fluid intake 2 hours before urine collection to avoid too great dilution of the parameters measured

- Urine can be kept at room temperature for up to 8 hours, and 24 hours in the refrigerator. It must not be frozen, but does not have to be at room temperature for the test

- When the test is positive, ovulation should take place within the next 24–36 hours. It is then useless to continue testing (it is preferable to keep the remaining tests, if needed, for the next cycle). Given that sperm is viable for 72 hours and ovum, for 12–24 hours, the maximum fertility period is from 2 days before ovulation to 1 day after

- The test cannot be reused

Table I: Calculation of Most Fertile Days
1. Calculate the length of menstrual cycles for 6–12 months
2. Subtract 18 days from the longest cycle and 11 days from the shortest cycle. This enables calculation of the first and last day of the most fertile period. For example, if the longest cycle is 38 days and the shortest cycle is 24 days, the fertile period is between the 13th and 20th day of the cycle (the first day being the first day of menstruation)

Table II: Advice for Maximizing Chances of Conception
1. Have sexual intercourse regularly, 2–3 times a week
2. When ovulation approaches, have sexual intercourse every day
3. Have a good lifestyle (eat well, exercise regularly, maintain a healthy weight)
4. Begin taking folic acid supplements 3 months before desired conception

When to consult

- If the woman tries to conceive during the most fertile period of each cycle for 6 menstrual cycles without success, a medical workup might be necessary

References

- Aikens Murphy A., Morgan K, Likis FE, Contraception. In:Durnell Schuiling K., Likis FE. Women's gynaecological health. 2005. Jones & Bartlett Ed. P. 169-219
- Alesksunes L. Optimizing conception through ovulation prediction. [Internet]. Drug store news 2005. [cited 2007 April 25]. Available from:http://www.firstresponse.com/ce/index.asp.
- Covington TR, et al. Nonprescription drug therapy: guiding patient self-care. 2nd edition. St-Louis: Facts & comparisons; 2003. p. 1302.
- Gaines D. Pros and cons of ovulation prediction kits [Internet]. Discovery.com. [cited 2007 April 25]. Available from: http://health.discovery.com/centers-pregnancy-americanbaby-opks.shtml.
- Mayo Clinic Staff. Pregnancy: how to get pregnant. [Internet]. Mayo Clinic.com: Tools for healthier lives. Mayo Foundation for Medical Education and Research. [cited 2007 November 13]. Available from: http://www.mayoclinic.com/health/how-to-get-pregnant/PR00103.
- Product monograph: First response. [Internet]. Church & Dwight Company. [cited 2007 April 27]. Available from: http://www.firstresponse.com/products/easyReadOvulationInsert.asp#use.

Pregnancy Tests

Pregnancy Tests

Overview

- The test is based on the detection of the β-hCG (human chorionic gonadotropin hormone) in the urine of pregnant women

- hCG is secreted by blastocyst cells, then by the placenta. It is composed of 2 subunits: α and β

- The OTC test uses monoclonal antibodies. A specific antibody links with the α chain, a chain also found in LH, FSH, and TSH, forming a complex along the control line

- A β-chain antibody is present and fixed on the "positive result" line, and this antibody links with β-hCG not forming a complex along the control line. The result is positive if there is a sufficient amount of β-hCG in urine

Questions to ask

✓ **When should the test be done?**

- ○ The test can be done up to 4 days before the expected menstruation date or 14 days after unprotected sex for women with irregular cycles or who are breastfeeding. **See Table I**

- ○ Ideally, the test should be done within 60–70 days of the delayed menstruation, because the level of β-hCG can decrease after this time

✓ **Presence of symptoms related to pregnancy?**

- ○ Increased breast tenderness

- ○ Increase in breast size

- ○ Darkening of areola

- ○ Nausea, vomiting, or both

- o Absence of menstruation or unusual menstruation (women can have blood with vaginal discharge or spotting during pregnancy)
- o Weight gain
- o Fatigue
- o Increase in urinary frequency

✓ **Time elapsed since sample taken and conservation method?**
  - o The urine sample can be kept in the refrigerator for up to 12 hours if the test cannot be done immediately
  - o It must, however, be at room temperature when the test is done, because urine that is too cold can result in a false negative

✓ **Medications taken by the patient?**
  - o Medications that increase secretion of LH and β-hCG such as *Pregnyl*, *Profasi*, *Pergonal*, *Metrodin*

✓ **Does the patient have any special conditions?**
  - o Ovarian cysts
  - o Ectopic pregnancy
  - o Recent delivery
  - o Recent miscarriage
  - o Spontaneous abortion in the past 8 weeks

What to do

If the patient wants to take the test at the pharmacy

- Ask the patient to take a urine sample. A morning sample (between 9:00 and 12:00) is preferable because the level of β-hCG is higher

If the patient wants to do the test at home

- Check the expiry date

- Do not use the urine sample if it is pink (or red), cloudy, or if you detect a strong or unusual odour

- Carefully read the manufacturer's instructions. Incorrect use of the test can lead to an incorrect result

- Comply with the required contact time between the urine and the stick, as well as the interval before taking a reading because they may vary depending on the test

- If the test chosen requires dipping a stick in a cup or directly in the urine stream, comply with the contact time in the instructions (use a stopwatch, watch, or timer)

- If the test chosen requires urine collection, use the cup that comes with the test and do not clean it with detergent because this could interfere with test results

- The first urine of the day (morning) has the highest concentration of β-hCG and its use may be recommended

- **If the test is positive** (positive if a line and control line appear, even if faint), there was sufficient β-hCG in the urine

- **If the test is negative**, the amount of β-hCG in the urine was insufficient to be detected. In these cases, the test can be repeated a few days later

- N.B.: Only a physician can diagnose or confirm pregnancy

- The test cannot be reused

Table I: Characteristics of Pregnancy Tests			
Name	Time Elapsed till Result (minutes)	Accuracy of Result (%)	Earliest Time to Do Test
One Step Pregnancy Test (S)	2	99	4 days before expected menstruation
Fact Plus (S)	2	99	4 days before expected menstruation
AccuClear (W)	1	99	N/A
First Response (S)	3	99	4 days before expected menstruation
Clearblue (S)	1	99	4 days before expected menstruation
OvuDate hCG	3	99	1st day period is late
Assure (S)	1 – 3	99	1st day period is late

S: stick, W: absorbent wick or pad

When to consult

- If the test is positive, make an appointment with an obstetrician/ gynecologist to ensure proper monitoring of the pregnancy

- If the test is negative after 2 more tests and if menstruation has not resumed

References

- Berry M. Pregnancy and fertility testing. Repchinsky C, Leblanc C, editors. Patient self-care: helping patients make therapeutic choices. 1st edition. Ottawa: Canadian Pharmacists Association; Welcom Ltd: 2002. p. 743-46
- Cossette B, Letarte N, Longtin J, et al. Étude comparative de neuf tests de grossesse offerts dans les pharmacies québécoises. Québec Pharmacie. 1996; 10:1043-48.
- Elizabeth E. How pregnancy tests work. [Internet]. HowThingsWork.com. [cited 2007 April 30]. Available from: http://health.howstuffworks.com/how-pregnancy-tests-work.htm.
- Martel M. Quels facteurs peuvent modifier le résultat d'un test de grossesse? Québec Pharmacie. 1995; 7:590 -91.
- Trupin SR, Valley V. Pregnancy. [Internet]. eMedecineHealth. [update 2005 October 08, cited 2007 April 30]. Available from: http://www.emedicinehealth.com/pregnancy/article_em.htm.

First-Aid Kits

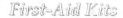
First-Aid Kits

Overview

- Keep in a dry, readily accessible place, known by everyone

- Keep in a place where injuries may happen or where the family spends a lot of time (e.g., car, cottage, house, boat, camping, on a trip, etc.)

- Metal or rigid plastic boxes are ideal (resist crushing, are water-resistant, preferably with separate compartments for orderly storage and quick access to the items needed)

- A first-aid kit must not replace care that may be required in more serious situations (e.g., extensive or deep wound or burn, bites by a wild animal whose history is unknown, eye injury, etc.). These serious cases require appropriate medical attention

What to use

Table I: Basic First-Aid Kit		
Pharmacy Items	**Medications**	**Other**
• Sterile gauze pads/rolls of various sizes (to apply to wounds, wash wounds, apply medications) • Adhesive tape to hold a gauze pad or bandage in place • Adhesive or nonadhesive bandages of various sizes • Elastic bandage • Instant cold compress • Bottle of saline solution (NaCl 0.9%) (to flush wounds) • 30 mL syringes with 19G needles (to flush wounds) • Isopropyl alcohol (70%) bottle or pads (clean instruments) • Disposable gloves • Eye patch	• Soap or antiseptic such as chlorhexidine or povidone-iodine (to wash hands and the skin around the wound) • Tube of <u>antibiotic cream</u> (to treat infected wounds) (e.g., gramicidin with polymyxin B) • Antibiotic drops for eyes/ears • Anti-H$_1$ oral antihistamines (e.g., diphenhydramine for allergic reactions) • Analgesic (e.g., acetaminophen/ ibuprofen) (for pain/fever)	• First-aid pocket book • Scissors • Pocket lamp (with new batteries) • Change (for pay phone) • List of emergency telephone numbers (police, anti-poison centre, family doctor, pharmacist, etc.) • Pencil/pen and sheets of paper • Splinter forceps • Moist towelettes to wipe wounds

Table II: Outdoor Kit		
Pharmacy Items	**Medications**	**Other**
· Bottles of insect repellent · Sunscreen (SPF≥ 30) · Sterile pad for a large wound · Elastic bandage for ankle/wrist · Liquid bandage (wounds not on flat surfaces, e.g., between fingers) · Thermometer	· Epinephrine loaded syringe, such as *EpiPen* or *Twinject* (if a family member has a history of severe allergy). Note the expiry date · Astringent (calamine lotion/cream without diphenhydramine) (for pruritus/redness due to insect bites) · Decongestant (e.g., pseudoephedrine) · Antidiarrhetic (e.g., loperamide) · Laxative (in suppository and oral form) · Tube of hydrocortisone 0.5% cream (pruritus, insect bites)	· **Basic First-Aid Kit** · Waterproof matches · Bottle of clove oil (for tooth pain) · Tincture of iodine (to purify water)

Table III: Travel Kit		
Pharmacy Items	**Medications**	**Other**
· Sunscreen (SPF ≥ 30) · **As well as some items from the Outdoor Kit**, according to destination	· Decongestant (e.g., pseudoephedrine) · Antidiarrhetic (e.g., loperamide) · Antiemetic (e.g., dimenhydrate) · Topical anesthetic · Astringent	· **Basic First-Aid Kit** · Tincture of iodine (to purify water)

Purifying Water with Iodine

Use this purification method only if it is impossible to boil water

- 5 drops of 2% tincture of iodine per litre of water (10 drops/L if water is very cold or opaque) or 12.5 mL of saturated iodine solution per litre of water (20mL/L if water is very cold or opaque) or 1 tablet of tetraglycine hydroperiodide per litre of water (2 tablets/litre if water is very cold or opaque)

- Let rest 30 minutes before consumption (a few hours if water is very cold or opaque), and at least 15 hours if possible presence of *Cryptosporidium* (water infestation by animal or human feces)

- It is essential to use the tincture because the regular solution is ineffective

- Prolonged use may be harmful

- To be avoided by **pregnant women** and individuals with **thyroid disorders**

References

- Berardi RR. Handbook of nonprescription drugs: an interactive approach to self-care. 15th edition. APhA; 2006.
- Canadian Pharmacists Association. Compendium of self-care products: the Canadian reference on OTCs. CPA; 2002-3.
- Desmarais N., Martineau J. La trousse de premiers soins (Part 1). Québec Pharmacie. 2007; 54:14-9.
- Ng H, Wong D. In: Repchinsky C, Leblanc C, editors. Patient self-care: helping patients make therapeutic choices. 1st edition. Ottawa: Canadian Pharmacists Association; Welcom Ltd: 2002. p. 834-44.
- Wolters Kluwer Health publishing group. Nonprescription drug therapy: guiding patient self-care. 5th edition. Wolters Kluwer; 2006. C1-C4.

Adjustment of Orthopedic

Devices

Crutches

- Wear flat shoes, stand straight, legs slightly apart
- Place the end of the crutch (lower end, with a rubber tip) about 15 cm from your foot
- Adjust the length of the crutches: there should be a space of two fingers between the armpit and the top of the crutch
- Adjustment of the hand grip: with arms at your sides, the hand grip should be at wrist level
- Using crutches
  - Do not lean your armpits on the top of the crutches
  - Transfer body weight to hands keeping the top part of the crutches firmly against the sides

Cane

- Wear flat shoes, stand straight, legs slightly apart
- Place the cane about 15 cm from your foot
- Adjustment of length of cane: with arms at your sides, the hand grip should be at wrist level
- Using a cane
  - When walking, hold the cane in the hand opposite the weak leg
  - Advance the cane at the same time as the weak leg
  - Push on the hand grip to move the other leg forward

Walker

- Wear flat shoes, stand straight, legs slightly apart
- Place the walker about 15 cm from your foot
- <u>Adjusting the height of the walker</u>: with arms at your sides, the hand grip on each side should be at wrist level
- <u>Using a walker</u>
  - Always slide the walker along the ground keeping the 4 legs in contact with the ground
  - Take a step
  - Push the 2 back legs of the walker to the level of the foot farthest ahead
  - Take another step and repeat

References

- Corporation professionnelle des physiothérapeutes du Québec. Comment ça marche? 1-16.

Immunization Schedule

Immunization Schedule

Overview

✓ Adhering to a regular schedule ensures the best possible protection

✓ Generally speaking, an interrupted vaccination series does not have to start over from the beginning, regardless of time elapsed

✓ In cases where a vaccination schedule was interrupted, a special age-appropriate schedule should be followed

Vaccination Schedules

Table I: Routine Vaccination Schedule									
Age at Time of Vaccination	DTaP-IPV	Hib	Var	MMR	d₂T₅/Tdap	HB	Pneu-C-7	Men-C	Other
Birth									
2 months	1	1				2	▨		
4 months	1	1					▨		
6 months	1	1				↑			1 [3]
12 months			4	5		or			
18 months	1	1		5					
4–6 years	5								
Pre-teen and teen years						7			
14–16 years					dCaT [8]				
50 years					9				
60 years									1 [10]
65 years									Pp

DTaP-IPV: Vaccine against diphtheria, tetanus, (acellular) pertussis combined with the inactivated poliomyelitis vaccine (*Quadracel*). *Pentacel* contains DTaP-IPV-Hib

Hib: Vaccine against *Haemophilus influenzae* type b (*Act-HIB*)

Var: Chickenpox vaccine (*Varivax III, Varilrix*)

MMR: Vaccine against measles, mumps, and rubella (*M-M-R II, Priotrix*)

d_2T_5: Diptheria and tetanus toxoid (for adults) (d_2T_5)

Tdap: Vaccine against diphtheria, tetanus, and (acellular) pertussis for adolescents and adults (*Adacel, Boostrix*)

HB: Hepatitis B vaccine (*Engerix-B, Recombivax HB*)

Pneu-C-7: Pneumococcal 7-valent conjugate vaccine (*Prevnar*)

Men-C: Meningococcal type C conjugate vaccine (*Menjugate, NeisVac-C, Meningitec*)

Inf: Influenza vaccine (traces of egg protein in *Fluviral, Vaxigrip*, and *Influvac* used in the 2006–2007 season). Caution, the influenza vaccination program and the vaccine compositions are renewed each autumn based on the probable strains in circulation

Pneu-P-23: Pneumococcal 23-valent polysaccharide vaccine (*Pneumovax 23, Pneumo 23*)

[1] Combined DTaP-Polio-Hib vaccine (*Pentacel*)

[2] Vaccination in 3 doses. If the mother is carrying the virus, the 1st dose should be given at birth. Otherwise, the 1st dose can be given at age 2 months. The 2nd dose should be given at least 1 month after the 1st dose. The 3rd dose should be given at least 2 months after the 2nd dose. In Canada, the preferred schedule is 0–1–6 months during the first year of life

[3] Recommended during the influenza (flu) season for all children age 6–23 months. For children under 9 years, administer 2 doses, 4 weeks apart, but the 2nd dose is not mandatory if the child was vaccinated the previous season

[4] Recommended for children age 12 months–12 years in a single dose. Administer on the 1st birthday, or as close as possible to that day. For children 13 and over, 2 doses ≥ 28 days apart

[5] Administer on the 1st birthday, or as close as possible to that day. It is recommended that a 2nd dose of MMR be administered ≥ 1 month after the 1st dose (better protection against measles)

[6] Combined DTaP-Polio vaccine (*Quadracel*). The dose can be omitted if the 4th dose of DTaP-IPV was administered after the 4th birthday

[7] Universal immunization against the hepatitis B virus is now part of the publicly funded vaccine programs offered in all provinces and territories. The age at which children and adolescents are offered HBV vaccine varies from jurisdiction to jurisdiction

8   Tdap for children ≥ 7 years. Then, d_2T_5 every 10 years. It should be noted that there is less diphtheria toxoid and pertussis antigen in the Tdap formulation than DTaP

9   It is recommended that the vaccination status be updated considering that most adults do not receive their booster shot every 10 years. Administer a single dose of Tdap if the person has never received an acellular pertussis, tetanus, and diphtheria vaccine

10   Administer annually

Table II: Person not Immunized According to the Regular Schedule (Child < 1 year)									
Appropriate Time for Vaccination	DTaP-IPV	Hib	Var	MMR	d_2T_5/Tdap	HB	Pneu-C-7	Men-C	Other
1st visit	1	1							
2 months later	1	1							
At ≥ 6 months									Inf [3]
At ≥ 12 months			4	5			11		
2 months after 2nd dose of DTaP	1	1, 12							
18 months									
12 months after 3rd dose of DTaP									
Continue with routine vaccination schedule									

11   Administer after the age of 1 year and at least 2 months after the 2nd dose. For children 7–11 months who are not immunized, the first 2 doses can be given ≥ 4 weeks apart

12   Omit this dose if the 1st dose was administered at age ≥ 7 months. In this case, administer the combined DTaP-Polio vaccine (*Quadracel*)

Table III: Person not Immunized According to the Routine Schedule (Child 1–6 years)								
Appropriate Time for Vaccination	DTaP-IPV	Hib	Var	MMR	d₂T₅ / Tdap	HB	Pneu-C-7	Men-C	Other
1st visit	1	1, 15		5			14		Inf [a]
2 months after 1st visit	1	1, 15		18			14, 17		
2 months after 2nd visit	16								
6-12 months after 3rd visit	19					.			
4–6 years	19								
Continue with routine vaccination schedule									

[13] If ≥ 5 years, primary vaccination against *Haemophilus influenzae* type b is not systematically recommended, can receive combined DCT-Polio vaccine (*Quadracel*)

[14] Omit if ≥ 5 years

[15] Omit if 1st dose administered at ≥ 15 months. In such a case, administer combined DCT-Polio vaccine (*Quadracel*)

[16] Administer this dose at ≥ 18 months

[17] Omit this dose if ≥ age 2 years when given the 1st dose, and in good health. Give 2nd dose in cases of chronic illness making the child susceptible to a pneumococcal infection

[18] Combined DCT-Polio vaccine (*Quadracel*)

[19] Not necessary if the 4th dose of DTaP or 3rd dose of IPV was given at ≥ age 4 years

Table IV: Person not Immunized According to the Regular Schedule (Child 7–17 years)						
Appropriate Time for Vaccination	d₂T₅/ TdaP	IPV	MMR	Var	Men-C	Other
1st visit	Tdap			20		
2 months after 1st visit	Tdap			4		HB [20,22]
6–12 months after 2nd visit	Tdap					
5–10 years after 3rd visit	D₂T₅ [21]					
Continue with routine vaccination schedule						

Men-C: Vaccine against meningococcus group C

[20] Booster for Var and HB given according to immunization protocol depending on jurisdiction

[21] Can be administered from age 14–16 respecting the 5-year period from the last dose of Tdap

[22] Give at 0–1–6 months during the first year of life

Table V: Person not Immunized According to the Routine Schedule (18 or older)						
Appropriate Time for Vaccination	**d₂T₅/ Tdap**	**IPV**	**MMR**	**Men-C**	**Var**	**Other**
1ˢᵗ visit	Tdap [23]	[23,24]	[24]			HB [22]
2 months later	d₂T₅ [25]	[24,25]	[24]		4	
6–12 months later	d₂T₅ [25,26]	[24,25]				
Continue with routine vaccination schedule						

[23] It is possible to administer a combined Tdap-Polio vaccine (*Adacel*)

[24] Should be offered to certain groups of adults (IPV: future parents or parents of young children; staff or student teachers at elementary and secondary schools, and at daycares; and to health-care workers [including trainees]. MMR: individuals considered as not vaccinated by one of the components)

[25] It is possible to administer a combined vaccine (*d₂T₅-Polio*)

[26] Then every 10 years

Table VI: Presence of Latex in Vaccines	
Boostrix [A]	*Typherix* [D]
Priorix [A]	*Avaxim 80* (80 antigen units) [E]
d₂T₅ [A]	*Imovax Rabies* [F]
Varilrix [A]	*Vaqta* [C]
Meningitec [C]	*Havrix* [D]
Recombivax HB [C]	*Menomune* [C]
Fluviral S/F [D]	*Pediacel* [C]
Prevnar [C]	*Pedvax HIB liquid* [C]
Pneumo 23 [E]	*Pentacel* [C]
YF-Vax [C]	*Quadracel* [C]
Typhim multi-dose vial	*Tripacel* [C]
Twinrix [D]	*TwinrixJunior* [D]

(A)   In the needle cap and the plunger of the syringe
(B)   In the stopper of the multi-dose vial
(C)   In the stopper of the vial
(D)   In the cap of pre-filled syringes
(E)   In the needle cap
(F)   In the vial cap vial and the plunger of the syringe

This section was adapted from the immunization protocol of Quebec and the Canadian Immunization Guide

<u>Vaccination and Travel</u>

- Consult a health-travel clinic or a family physician 2–3 months before departure

Table VII: Specific Vaccines for Travellers		
	Vaccines	**Indications**
Basic Vaccine	**Diptheria and tetanus toxoid**	For travel to developing countries where tetanus toxoid cannot be safely administered. An advanced booster shot can be given if the last dose was received more than 5 years ago
		Booster shots recommended every 10 years
	Poliomyelitis vaccine	All travellers should be vaccinated
		IPV booster shot for adults if the person is travelling in a polio-endemic or epidemic region
	Vaccine against measles, mumps, and rubella—adult	MMR (preferably) if the person was born in or after 1970 and is traveling to a measles-endemic area, unless there is serological proof of immunity or physician documentation of prior measles
		Protection against rubella is especially important for women of childbearing age who are not immune
	Vaccine against measles, mumps, and rubella—infants and children	For travel to a measles-endemic region
		MMR can be given as early as 6 months of age, but then the routine series of 2 doses must still be restarted after the child is 12 months old
	Hepatitis B vaccine—adults (*Engerix-B* and *Recombivax HB*)	Not previously vaccinated and traveling to and residing > 6 months in areas with high levels of endemic hepatitis B
		Not previously vaccinated and working in health-care facilities
		Not previously vaccinated and likely to have contact with blood or to have sexual contact with residents of areas with high levels of endemic hepatitis B
	Hepatitis B vaccine—infants and children (*Engerix-B* and *Recombivax HB*)	Children of any age who will live in an area where hepatitis B is endemic should receive full hepatitis B immunization

Table VII: Specific Vaccines for Travellers (cont'd)		
	Vaccines	**Indications**
Required Vaccines	**Yellow fever vaccine** (*YF-Vax*)	Required age: 9 months or older
		Traces of egg protein in *YF-Vax*
		People who go to places where cases have been officially reported (Africa or South America) or travelling in areas where the illness is endemic
		The only vaccine that can be mandatory for entry into certain countries by virtue of the International Health Regulations of the WHO
		A list of travel clinics that can offer a vaccination certificate for yellow fever can be found at the Public Health Agency of Canada's Travel Medicine Program at www.travelhealth.gc.ca
	Cholera vaccine (*Mutacol-oral*) (*Dukoral-oral*) also against enterotoxigenic *E. coli* diarrhea)	Required age: 2 years or older
		May be required by certain local authorities
		Certain travel clinics provide a cholera "exemption certificate" which is used to help travellers avoid being given cholera vaccine while abroad
		Infection avoidable through precaution when eating Oral rehydration treatment is effective
		In some cases, should be considered if staying in endemic or epidemic areas under inadequate sanitary conditions

Table VII: Specific Vaccines for Travellers (cont'd)		
	Vaccines	**Indications**
Recommended Vaccines	**Hepatitis A vaccine** (*Havrix, Vaqta, Avaxim, Epaxal Berna*)	Required age: ≥ 1 year (*Havrix, Avaxim, Epaxal Berna*), ≥ 2 years (*Vaqta*)
		Highly recommended for travellers going to developing countries
		If contraindicated or < 1 year, administer immunoglobulins immediately before departure for 4–6 months' protection
		Epaxal Berna cross-allergy with vaccine against influenza
	Typhoid vaccine (*Typhim Vi, Typherix*) (*Vivotif Berna L-oral* (liquid), *Vivotif Berna-oral* [capsules])	Required age: injectable→2 years or older, oral→ 3 years or older
		Prolonged exposure (> 4 weeks) to potentially contaminated food and water. Not routinely recommended for business travel or short-term (< 4 weeks) holidays in resort hotels
		Individuals ≥ 2 years in close, constant contact with a carrier of *Salmonella typhi*
		Laboratory employees handling cultures of *Salmonella typhi*
	Vaccine against meningococcus (adult) *Menjugate, NeisVac-C, Meningitec, Menactra*)	Long stay in a region where incidence of infection is high
		Optional for short-term travellers (< 3 weeks) on business or holidays if little contact with the local population. Consider vaccination even if the stay is < 3 weeks if there will be close contact with the local population in endemic areas; if there will be travel to epidemic areas; or, if the traveller will be providing health care to others
		Proof of menigococcal immunization is required for entry into Saudi Arabia for pilgrims travelling to Mecca during the Hajj
	Vaccine against meningococcus— infants and children	To travel to regions where broader protection is needed, consider vaccinating children 2 months or older (*Menjugate, NeisVac-C, Meningitec*)

Table VII: Specific Vaccines for Travellers (cont'd)		
Vaccines		**Indications**
Recommended Vaccines	**Japanese encephalitis vaccine** (*JE-Vax*)	Required age: 1 year or older
		Trip where the traveller will spend at least 4 weeks in endemic or epidemic areas during the transmission season
		Plan on having the vaccine even if stay is < 4 weeks in an endemic region and if extensive outdoor rural exposure
	Rabies vaccine (*Imovax Rabies*) (*RabAvert*)	Pre-exposure immunization according to personal risk (e.g., veterinarians, people who handle potentially rabid animals, travellers to areas at risk, etc.)
		Pre-exposure vaccination does not eliminate the necessity of post-exposure vaccination
		It is recommended to start treatment within 24 hours of exposure, but there is no limit beyond which prophylaxis is no longer recommended
		Cultivated in chicken embryonic cells (caution in case of egg allergy, but no contraindication with regard to the use of a post-exposure vaccine)
	Influenza vaccine	People at risk of complications from influenza who are preparing to travel to a country where the virus is probably present
		Use the most recent vaccine
	Tuberculosis vaccine (*BCG*)	For infants and children who will be staying in areas where there is a high risk of infection (> 1%/year), in case of high risk of illness after contact, and for children ≥ 5 years staying for extended periods in areas at risk
		For health-care workers at high risk of exposure to tuberculosis bacillus

Table VII: Specific Vaccines for Travellers (cont'd)		
	Vaccines	**Indications**
Recommended Vaccines	**European tick-borne encephalitis vaccine** (*FSME-IMMUN*)	Required age: 16 years or older
		Long stay in an endemic region, with frequent, prolonged activities in grassy or wooded areas
		Not authorized in Canada, but may be obtained through the HPB Special Access Program; in Austria; or in health-travel clinics in London, England. Contact IMMUNO-CANADA at 1 800 551-0478
		Cultivated in chicken embryonic cells (caution in case of egg allergy)
	Rotavirus vaccine (*RotaTeq*) (oral)	Infants 6–32 weeks
		Against severe acute gastroenteritis
		Recently approved in Canada, but not yet approved for routine administration in Canada
		Can be administered to infants with a prior rotavirus infection
	Human Papilloma Virus vaccine (HPV) (*Gardasil*)	Not yet approved for routine administration in Canada
		For girls and women age 9–26 years, ideally at the beginning of sexual activity
		Can be administered even if the person has already had an HPV infection because the immunity acquired is specific to type

This section was adapted from the immunization protocol of Quebec and the Canadian Immunization Guide

A listing of travel clinics across Canada can be found online at www.travelhealth.gc.ca

References

- Public Health Agency of Canada, Infectious Disease and Emergency Preparedness Branch and Center for Infectious Disease Prevention and Control under the Authority of the Minister of Public Works and Governement Services of Canada. Canadian Immunization Guide. 7th edition; 2006. [Internet]. Canada. [cited 2007 April 01]. Available from: http://www.phac-aspc.gc.ca/publicat/cig-gci/pdf/cig-gci-2006_e.pdf.
- Ministère de la Santé et des Services sociaux. Chapters 6–14. In: Protocole d'immunisation, 4th edition. Québec: La Direction des communications du ministère de la Santé et des Services sociaux; 2004. p. 105-342N. [Internet]. Quebec. [cited 2007 April 01]. Available from: www.msss.gouv.qc.ca.
- Anonymous. Travel Health: Know before you go! [Internet]. Public Health Agency of Canada. [cited 2007 April 1]. Available from: www.travelhealth.gc.ca.

Pre-surgery Medication

Pre-surgery Medication

- Before surgery, the relevance of some medications should be re-evaluated, either because the patient must comply with the directive "nil per os" as closely as possible, or because some medications can complicate surgery

- Where there is doubt, hospitals often have pharmacists who are experienced in adjusting pre-surgery medications

- Generally speaking, personnel of the surgical care unit have specific pre- and post-surgery medication protocols

- The directives suggested here apply only in general cases, and adjustments must often be made to certain steps depending on the patient's health and according to the surgeon's instructions

Table I: Pre-operatory Directives	
Medications	**Directives**
Coagulation	
Acetylsalicylic acid (ASA)	Irreversibly inhibits platelet function; patient must stop taking it at least 7 days before surgery. Do not discontinue ASA if patient has a history of myocardial infarction
Nonsteroidal antinflammatory drugs (NSAIDs)	Discontinue before elective surgery because these can increase the risk of postoperative bleeding Consider 5 times half-life in regard to the time to stop before surgery
Clopidogrel	Stop at least 5 (preferably 7) days before surgery
Ticlopidine	Stop at least 7–14 days before surgery
Warfarin	Stop 2–5 days until the INR is below 1.5. Administration of Vitamin K may be necessary the day of surgery. Heparin often serves as a pre- and post-operative back-up

Table I: Pre-operatory Directives (cont'd)	
Medications	**Directives**
Central Nervous System	
Alcohol	Chronic use can increase needs in anesthesia while acute intoxication reduces needs in anesthesia
	Caution with withdrawal symptoms
Narcotics	Continue until surgery
	Withdrawal symptoms possible if surgery is long or if the dose is insufficient
Tricyclic antidepressants	Often uninterrupted. However, many interactions, long half-life, proarrhythmic effect requires certain precautions for the choice of anesthetic
Serotonin reuptake inhibitors	Continue because there is risk of withdrawal syndrome
Venlafaxine	Wise to interrupt administration 24–48 hours before surgery (risk of hypertension and paroxystic tachycardia with vasopressors) Consult treating psychiatrist
Endocrinology	
Corticosteroid therapy	Adjusted in hospital environment. Continued for most patients (especially asthmatics)
Oral hypoglycemic agents	Stop the morning of surgery
	Insulin therapy is usually initiated during hospitalization
Insulin	Insulin will be continued but the regimen modified
Estrogens	Stop the morning of surgery
Oral contraceptives	Stop one month before surgery for patients undergoing major surgery and who are at high risk for thrombosis
Cardiovascular System Medications	
Statins	Continue (improved prognosis after vascular surgery)
Beta-blockers	Continue (because withdrawal increases the risk of ischemic events and mortality)
Angiotensin-converting enzyme inhibitors (ACEIs) and angiotensin receptor antagonists (ARBs)	Stop the night before because there is a risk of hypotension
Calcium channel blockers	Continue (rebound effect if stopped)

Table I: Pre-operatory Directives (cont'd)	
Medications	**Directives**
Diuretics	Stop the morning of surgery (re: hypovolemia, metabolic anomalies) (will be adjusted by medical team during surgery)
α2-agonists	Continue (rebound effect if stopped)
Class I antiarrhythmic drugs	Given their proarrhythmogenic effect, suggest they be stopped but at the risk of seeing the rhythmic anomaly reappear (atrial fibrillation or flutter). To be discussed with the surgeon and cardiologist
Class III antiarrhythmic drugs	To be discussed with the surgeon and cardiologist. Beware of QT interval prolongation
Amiodarone	Continue until the morning of surgery. Long half-life makes stopping difficult. Poses few problems in practice
Digoxin	Generally not discontinued. Important to have a level the morning of surgery. Careful if hypokalemia, acidosis, and renal failure
Gastrointestinal System Medications	
H_2-receptor antagonists	Will be administered pre-op in many types of surgeries
Antacids in suspension	Not recommended because of the risk of pulmonary damage if aspiration
Prokinetic agents (e.g., domperidone, metoclopramide)	If given 1–2 hours pre-op will ensure better gastric emptying, especially for diabetics
For inflammatory bowel disease	Continue administration before the operation
Vitamins and Supplements	
Multivitamins	Stop the morning of surgery
Iron	Stop the morning of surgery
Natural products	In general, stop at least 2–3 weeks before surgery
Echinacea	Stop (decreases efficacy of immunosuppressors)
Ephedra	Stop at least 24 hours before surgery
Garlic	Stop at least 7 days before surgery
Gingko biloba	Stop at least 36 hours before surgery
Ginseng	Stop at least 7 days before surgery
Kava kava, St. John's Wort, valerian	Withdraw over a few days. For St. John's Wort, stop at least 5 days before surgery

Table I: Pre-operatory Directives (cont'd)	
Medications	**Directives**
Other	
Bronchodilator	Use it up to time of surgery so as to maximize pulmonary function
Antihistamines	Continue
Antitussives/ Decongestants	Stop with surgery
	If the patient has a respiratory infection, the timing of surgery should be reassessed

These tables are not comprehensive. Some classes of medications are not discussed given that they depend more on the patient's condition

References

- Stafford Smith M, Muir H, Hall R. Perioperative management of drug therapy. Clinical Considerations. Drugs. 1996; 51:238-259.
- Antman EM, Anbe DT, Armstrong PW, et al. ACC/AHA guidelines for the management of patients with ST-elevation myocardial infarction-- executive summary. A report of the American College of Cardiology/American Heart Association Task Force on Practice Guidelines (Writing Committee to revise the 1999 guidelines for the management of patients with acute myocardial infarction). J Am Coll Cardiol. 2004; 44:671-719.
- Tirumalasetty J, Grammer LC. Asthma, surgery, and general anesthesia: a review. J Asthma. 2006; 43:251-4.
- C. Baillard. Conduite à tenir concernant le traitement médicamenteux des patients adressés pour chirurgie programmée. Ann Fr Anesth Reanim. 2005; 24:1360-74.
- Ottawa SM, Ramuscak N. Pre- and postoperative care of surgical patients. Pharmacy Practice. 1996.
- Doak GJ. Discontinuing drugs before surgery. Canadian Journal of anesthesia 1997; 44:R112-17.
- Villeneuve, Maude. Quels sont les agents affectant l'hémostase en période périopératoire? Québec Pharmacie. 2005; 52: 296-9.
- Ang-Lee MK, Moss J, Yuan CS, Herbal Medicines and Perioperative Care. JAMA. 2001; 286: 208-16.

Chronic Renal Failure
and OTC Medication

Overview

- Avoid major fluid intake if there is a fluid restriction

- Avoid all products too high in electrolytes (e.g., sodium biphosphate, milk of magnesia)

- Given that this population uses multiple medications, be careful of drug-drug and drug-disease interactions

- Given the frequent contact with a physician and the complexity of disorders related to chronic renal failure (CRF), it is suggested that patients discuss every health problem with a physician

Table I: Directives for Using Medications in Chronic Renal Failure		
Problem	**Use**	**Avoid**
Gastrointestinal Disorders		
Constipation	<u>Good choice</u> Docusate sodium or calcium (Polyethylene glycol: small daily quantity) Lactulose <u>Occasional use</u> Glycerin suppositories Mineral oil enema Mineral oil, orally Sennoside or bisacodyl Cascara sagrada[5]	Soluble fibre[1] Increase in dietary fibre[1] Major water intake[1] Oral laxatives or sodium biphosphate-based laxatives[2] Magnesium hydroxide[3] Magnesium citrate[2] Other saline laxatives Natural products[4] Licorice Rhubarb

Table I: Directives for Using Medications in Chronic Renal Failure (cont'd)		
Problem	**Use**	**Avoid**
Diarrhea/ flatulence	Stop/reduce constipation medication Soluble fibres Loperamide Simethicone	Bismuth salts Attapulgite Major rehydration[1]
Nausea/ vomiting	Dimenhydrinate	Major rehydration[1]
Dyspepsia	Ranitidine* Famotidine*	Aluminum or magnesium hydroxide[3] Calcium carbonate[3] Sodium bicarbonate[3] Other saline anti-acids
Cold/Flu		
Congestion	Nasal spray 0.9% NaCl Topical pediatric decongestant Topical camphor Eucalyptus oil (topical)	Pseudoephedrine[9] po Ammonium chloride
Fever	Acetaminophen	ASA[6] NSAIDs[7]
Sore throat	Acetaminophen	ASA[6] NSAIDs[7]
Cough	Dextromethorphan[8] Exempted codeine[8]* Guaifenesin	
Pain	Acetaminophen Topical analgesics Topical anti-irritants	ASA[6] NSAIDs[7] Exempted codeine[8] Methyl salicylate
Allergic rhinitis	Loratadine* Cetirizine* Fexofenadine* Desloratadine* Diphenhydramine* po Chlorpheniramine	

Table I: Directives for Using Medications in Chronic Renal Failure (cont'd)		
Problem	**Use**	**Avoid**
Pruritus	<u>General</u> Topical emollient Colloidal oatmeal Diphenhydramine* po <u>Localized/limited area</u> Topical hydrocortisone Capsaicin-based cream Anti-irritants Topical anesthetics	Topical antihistamines
Minerals/ vitamins	Vitamin D_{10} Zinc[11]	
Ophthalmic problems	Hypromellose Polyethylene glycol Tetrahydrozoline	

[1]   To be avoided only if fluid restriction

[2]   Absolute contraindication

[3]   Not absolutely contraindicated. Can lead to an electrolytic imbalance and/or an accumulation of aluminum

[4]   Accumulation of products and their contaminants unknown in chronic renal failure

[5]   Use with caution. Can interact with diuretics. Long-term use can cause hypokalemia

[6]   Not absolutely contraindicated. Use low dose to prevent cardiovascular disease

[7]   Not absolutely contraindicated if light to moderate failure, but limit use as much as possible so as to preserve renal function as long as possible. Can cause interstitial nephritis, nephrotic syndrome, papillary necrosis, membranous nephropathy, and hypertension

[8]   Not absolutely contraindicated, but significant risk of accumulation of metabolites causing major adverse effects

[9]   Can cause hypertension

[10] Not absolutely contraindicated, but can cause hypercalcemia and a hypervitaminosis D

[11] Possible accumulation, therefore, do not use continuously

*   Can be administered but moderate dosage adjustment necessary

References

- Lacy CF, Armstrong LL, Goldman MP, Lance LL. Drug information handbook. 15th edition. Hudson: Lexi-Comp; 2007.
- Laliberté M-C, Normandeau M, Lord A, Lamarre D, Cantin I, Berbiche D, Corneille L, Prud'homme L, Lalonde L. Use of over-the-counter medications and natural products in patients with moderate and severe chronic renal insufficiency. Am J Kidney Dis. 2007; 49: 245-256.
- Aronoff GR, Berns JS, Brier ME, Golper TA, Morrison G, Singer I, Swan SK, Benett WM. Drug prescribing in renal failure: Dosing guidelines for adults. 4th edition. Philadelphia: American College of Physicians; 1999.
- Moore GD, Klasco R, editors. Dosing & therapeutic tools database. [Internet]. MICROMEDEX, Greenwood Village, Colorado. [cited 2003 November 1]. Available from: http://healthcare.micromedex.com.
- Lord A, Ménard C. Médicaments en vente libre, produits naturels et insuffisance rénale. Le Médecin du Québec. 2002; 37: 61-6.
- Lord A, Ménard C. La néphrotoxicité médicamenteuse: comment limiter les dégâts? Le médecin du Québec. 2002; 37:55-9.
- Fitzgerald J. Narcotic analgesic in renal failure. Connecticut Medecine. 1991; 55:701-4.
- Schwartz IF, Iaina A. Uraemis pruritus. Nephrol Dial Transplant. 1999; 14:834-9.
- Tarng DC, Cho YL, Liu HN, Huang TP. Hemodialysis-related pruritus: a double-blind, placebo-controlled, crossover study of capsaicine 0.025% cream. Néphron. 1996; 72: 617-22.
- Millikan LE. Treating pruritus: what's new in safe relief of symptoms? Postgrad Med. 1996; 99:173-84.

Vitamins, Minerals,
and Nutritional Supplements

- The problems dealt with in this chapter are presented in the following order:
  - o Iron deficiency anemia
  - o Scar healing
  - o Osteoporosis
  - o Prevention of isoniazid-induced neuropathy
  - o Prevention of spina bifida
  - o Premenstrual syndrome
  - o Precautions and contraindications

Iron deficiency anemia

- Dose for treatment of iron deficiency anemia: 180 mg of elemental iron per day

Table I: Elemental Iron Content		
Iron salt	Mg/tablet	Elemental iron/tablet
Ferrous sulfate	300	60
Ferrous gluconate	300	35
Ferrous fumarate	200	66

- Advice regarding iron intake:
  - o Preferably taken on an empty stomach (if not tolerated, take with a small amount of food)
  - o Take with orange juice (or another acid beverage)
  - o Can cause black stools
  - o Liquid form can stain teeth

- o Iron requires an acid environment to be absorbed; a patient under antacid treatment (PPI, H_2-receptor antagonist) will not absorb iron as well. Concomitantly taking 200 mg or more of Vitamin C per 30 mg of elemental iron may increase absorption

Scar Healing

- Topical Vitamin E: contradictory data
- Vitamin E po: 200–400 mg per day for 3–4 months (a study with 57 subjects suggests accelerated healing, but these are very limited data)

Osteoporosis

Table II: Osteoporosis and Daily Calcium Intake	
Age	Elemental Ca Intake (mg per day)
9–12	1300
19–50	1000
50 +	1000–1500

- Do not take more than 500 mg per dose to maximize calcium absorption
- Dose of Vitamin D for prevention or treatment of osteoporosis: 400–800 IU/day

Prevention of isoniazid-induced neuropathy

- Vitamin B_6: 10–50 mg per day
- Note: Any patient taking isoniazid must take a Vitamin B supplement

Prevention of spina bifida in newborns

- Any woman of childbearing age should, in principle, take a 0.4 mg/day supplement of folic acid
- It is recommended to start taking folic acid at least 3 months before pregnancy and to continue for at least the first 3 months of pregnancy

| Table III: Dosage of Folic Acid in Pregnant Women to Prevent Congenital Malformations ||
Specific Cases	Recommended Dosage
Diabetic (type 1 and 2)	1–5 mg
Under treatment with an anticonvulsant (valproic acid, carbamazepine, phenytoin)	
History of pregnancy with neural tube anomaly	5 mg

Premenstrual syndrome

| Table IV: Agents that May Help in Premenstrual Syndrome |||
Agent	Dosage	Comments
Vitamin B6	50–100 mg per day	Can reduce the symptoms of premenstrual syndrome
Elemental calcium	1200 mg per day	Greater efficacy than a placebo in reducing pain and water retention and managing increased appetite and bad mood

Precautions/contraindications

- Pregnancy
  - Do not exceed the recommended daily intake for Vitamin A and carotenoids (800 RE)
- 1 RE = 1 µg retinol
  - = 6 µg beta carotene
  - = 3.3 IU retinol
  - = 9.9 IU beta carotene
- Patient treated with warfarin
  - **Vitamin E** in the amount of 800 IU or more per day can increase INR. Avoid Vitamin E supplements if possible
  - The amount of Vitamin E contained in multivitamins should not cause an interaction

- Interactions
  - Multivitamins can bind to certain medications (e.g., ciprofloxacin) and decrease absorption
  - Suggest taking multivitamins 1–2 hours after any medication that may be chelated by minerals

References

- Beveridge C. Basic nutrition. In: Repchinsky C, Leblanc C, editors. Patient self-care: helping patients make therapeutic choices. 1st edition. Ottawa: Canadian Pharmacists Association; Welcom Ltd: 2002. p. 340-358.
- Brown TER, Campbell C. Dysmenorrhea and premenstrual syndrome. In: Repchinsky C, Leblanc C, editors. Patient self-care: helping patients make therapeutic choices. 1st edition. Ottawa: Canadian Pharmacists Association; Welcom Ltd: 2002. p. 684-694.
- Ferreira E. Acide folique et la prévention des anomalies de tube neural. Québec Pharmacie. 2000; 47: 726-30.
- Gagné-Tremblay ME. Produits pour diminuer l'apparence des cicatrices. Québec Pharmacie. 2001; 48:315-18.
- Lacy CF, Armstrong LL, Goldman MP, Lance LL. Drug information handbook. 8th edition. American Pharmaceutical Association. Lexi-Comp; 2000-2001.

Malnutrition and
Nutritional Supplements

Overview

- Definition: Malnutrition occurs when caloric or protein intake is insufficient to meet the requirements of the organism
- Signs and symptoms:
  - At the beginning: drop in energy, overall weakness, apathy, weight loss, weight loss with loss of subcutaneous fat
  - Later: decrease in muscular mass, absence of subcutaneous fat, dryness, thinning and change in texture of hair. Decrease in heart rate, blood pressure, and body temperature is also possible
- Complications: weight loss, loss of visceral proteins, decreased immunity, poor scarring ability, decrease in functional skill and strength

Questions to ask

- ✓ **What are your dietary habits?**
  - Several meetings and keeping a journal documenting the type and quantity of food ingested may be necessary
- ✓ **Have you noticed any change in the nature/appearance of your hair, eyes, face, teeth, gums, skin, or nails?**
  - Denotes a vitamin and/or mineral deficiency accompanying malnutrition
- ✓ **Have you noticed that your wounds take longer to heal?**
- ✓ **Have you noticed a weight change?**
- ✓ **Have you noticed a decrease in your functional skills, in your level of strength or energy?**
- ✓ **Do you drink alcohol or take illicit drugs?**

✓ **Have you had any health problems lately?**

✓ **Do you have any chronic diseases? What is the severity of these diseases?**

- o Chronic obstructive pulmonary disease (COPD), hepatic failure, heart failure, diabetes, inflammatory bowel disease, etc.

What to do

Prevention

- Follow the recommendations of the latest version of Canada's Food Guide
- The number of portions in each food group varies based on sex and age group

Table I: Canada's Food Guide Recommended Number of Servings per Day				
	19–50 years		**51 years or older**	
	Females	**Males**	**Females**	**Males**
Vegetables and Fruit	7–8	8–10	7	7
Grain products	6–7	8	6	7
Milk and alternatives	2	2	3	3
Meat and alternatives	2	3	2	3
Unsaturated fat	30–45 mL			

Adapted from Health Canada, Canada's Food Guide

Some patient populations may need a diet adapted to their state of health (e.g., renal failure, diabetes) and a dietetics consultation may be necessary

Treatment

- Steps to follow in choosing the type and quantity of supplements/food substitutes adapted to a given person

1. Evaluate a person's daily energy requirements

Table II: Schofield Equations		
Male	18–30 years	15.1 (weight in kg) + 692.2
	30–60 years	11.5 (weight in kg) + 873.1
	> 60 years	11.7 (weight in kg) + 587.7
Female	18–30 years	14.8 (weight in kg) + 486.6
	30–60 years	8.1 (weight in kg) + 845.6
	> 60 years	9.1 (weight in kg) + 658.5

Adapted from *Food and Agricultural Organization, Human Energy Requirements*

- Energy requirements = basic requirements x level of physical activity
  - Level of physical activity
    - Sedentary or slightly active person: 1.40–1.69
    - Active or moderately active person: 1.70–1.99
    - Very active person: 2.00–2.40
  - A level of activity above 2.40 is difficult to maintain over the long term

2. Assessment of individual carbohydrate, protein, fat, and fibre requirements

Table III: The Breakdown of Sources of Energy Varies by Age Group			
	Percentage of Total Calories from		
Age group	Carbohydrates (4 cal/g)	Proteins (4 cal/g)	Fat (9 cal/g)
1–3 years	45–65%	2–20%	30–40%
4–18 years	45–65%	10–30%	25–35%
19 years or older	45–65%	10–35%	20–35%

- Recommended daily fibre intake: 14 g per 1000 calories
- Recommended fluid intake: 1 mL per calorie or 30 mL/kg
- The breakdown of sources of energy and other requirements can vary based on the person's state of health

What to use

- There are various supplement/meal substitute formulations on the market, many of them offered without a prescription

Table IV: Characteristics of Different Types of Formulations (non-exhaustive list)		
Polymeric	Proteins: intact Fats: intact Carbohydrates: polymers	Provide complete nutrition Used orally or by tube Suitable for most patients
Oligomeric	Proteins: hydrolized or partially hydrolized Fats: long- or medium-chain triglycerides Carbohydrates: partially hydrolized or oligosaccharides	Used in case of digestive disorders or malabsorption (pancreatic failure, short-intestine syndrome)
Modular	A single macroelement Proteins, fats, or carbohydrates	Added to food or to other food supplements To increase caloric or protein intake
Increased branched-chain amino acid content	↑ leucine, isoleucine, and valine ↓ tryptophan, tyrosine et phenylalanine (aromatic amino acids)	Used in case of hepatic failure or hepatic encephalopathy Used in case of severe stress accompanied by multiple organ failure or dysfunction (sepsis, severe trauma)
Increased essential amino acid content	↑ leucine, isoleucine, valine + histidine	Used in case of renal failure, sepsis, or trauma
With fibre	Content varies from 6–14 g/1000 calories	Not suitable for a residue-reduced diet Helps maintain intestinal regularity

Table IV: Characteristics of Different Types of Formulations (non-exhaustive list) (cont'd)		
Caloric density	1 calorie/mL	General population requiring a food supplement
	1.5 calorie/mL	Population requiring limited volume energy and protein intake
	2 calories/mL	Population requiring a limited volume energy and protein intake
		Risk of dehydration and electrolytic anomalies
Lactose free		Used in case of lactose intolerance
		Polymeric and oligomeric formulations are lactose free
For diabetics	50% of calories are in the form of fats, of which 70% are in the form of monounsaturated fatty acids	*Glucerna* significantly reduces the increase in glycemia in type 1 and 2 diabetes, compared with other formulations
	35% of calories are in the form of carbohydrates	
	Carbohydrates (maltodextrin, fructose, soy polysaccharides) prevent the rapid absorption of glucose	
For patients with hepatic failure	Increased branched-chain amino acid (BCAA) content (leucine, isoleucine et valine)	The AAAs act as false neurotransmitters to the brain and contribute to hepatic encephalopathy
	Reduced aromatic amino acid (AAA) content (tryptophan, tyrosine, phenylalanine)	Modest effect in the treatment of hepatic encephalopathy not demonstrated in higher quality studies
		Seems to reduce the frequency of complications and to increase nutritional status in the presence of cirrhosis

Table IV: Characteristics of Different Types of Formulations (non-exhaustive list) (cont'd)		
For patients with renal failure	Reduced protein content ↑ ratio essential amino acids (EAAs)/non-essential amino acids (NEAAs) Formulation for dialysis patients, richer in protein than for non-dialysis patients Reduced electrolytic content Absence of vitamins Higher caloric density	A reduced-protein diet slows progression of the disease in the non-dialysis population The ↑ ratio of EAA/NEAA aims at reducing the metabolic load (e.g., urea) that the kidney can no longer eliminate
For chronic obstructive pulmonary disease (COPD)	Increased fat and reduced carbohydrate content 50% of calories in the form of fats	Combustion of fats requires less O_2 and produces less CO_2 than combustion of carbohydrates The benefits are not clinically significant for most patients. Patients with borderline respiratory function benefit more
For inflammatory bowel diseases	Oligomeric macroelements	These formulations are less allergenic, but no difference has been noted when they are compared with polymer formulations
Other specialized formulations	Composition adapted based on a genetic deficit	Absence of phenylalanine
Other characteristics	Osmolality 270–700 mOsm/kg of water	Osmolality increases with caloric density and oligomeric formulations Higher incidence of diarrhea by drawing water with osmolality > 300 mOsm/kg water
	Kosher	Ross, a division of Abbott Laboratories makes kosher formulations
	Gluten free	Used in case of celiac disease (gluten intolerance)

- Advice to patients
  - Once opened, food supplement containers should be kept in the refrigerator and used within 24 hours so as to avoid bacterial contamination

When to consult

- Presence of comorbidities (COPD, renal failure, hepatic failure, heart failure, diabetes, etc.)
- In the presence of severe malnutrition (prolonged fasting, anorexia, cachexia, etc.)
- Pregnant or breastfeeding woman
- Person under 18
- Person who would like to eat only supplements for more than 24 hours

References

- Butte NF, Caballero B. Energy needs: Assessment and requirements. In: Shils ME, Shike M, Ross AC, Caballero B, Cousins JR. Modern nutrition in health and disease. 10th edition. Baltimore: Lippincott Williams & Wilkins; 2006. p. 136-148.
- Cano NJ, Fouque D, Leverve XM. Application of branched-chain amino acids in human pathological states: Renal failure. J Nutr. 2006; 136:299-307.
- Charlton M. Branched-chain amino acid enriched supplements as therapy for liver disease. J Nutr. 2006; 136:295-8.
- Facts and comparisons. Nutrition. In: Nonprescription drug therapy: guiding patient self-care. 5th edition. St-Louis: Facts and comparisons; 2006. p. 217-254.
- Food and Agriculture Organization, World Health Organization, United National University. Report of a joint FAO/WHO/UNU expert consultation: human energy requirements. Food and nutrition technical report series 1. Rome: FAO, 2001.
- Koretz RL, Avenell A, Lipman TO, Braunshweig CL, Miline AC. Does enteral nutrition affect clinical outcome? A systematic review of the randomized trials. Am J Gastroenterol. 2007;102:412-429.

- Laboratoires Abbott, Limitée. Guide des aliments thérapeutiques: composition, utilisation, saveurs et formats, caractéristiques nutritionnelles. [Internet]. In: Laboratoires Abbott, Limitée. Principaux secteurs thérapeutiques. Alimentation. Adultes. [cited 2007 May 03]. Available from: https://abbott.ca/fr/images/health/content/inter.pdf.
- Novartis Nutrition Canada. Full product list. [Internet]. Novartis Consumer Health Canada Ltd. [cited 2007 May 07]. Available from: http://www.novartisnutrition.com/ca/productList.
- Rollin CJ. Functional and meal replacement foods. Dans: Berardi RR, Kroon LA, McDermott JH, Newton GD, Oszko MA, Popovich NG, et al, editors. Handbook of nonprescription drugs: an interactive approach to self-care. 15th edition. Washington: American Pharmacists Association; 2006. p. 475-502.
- Health Canada. Eating well with Canada's food guide. Health Canada: Food and Nutrition. [cited 2007 May 03]. Available from: http://www.hc-sc.gc.ca/fn-an/food-guide-aliment/index_e.html. Shike M. Enteral feeding. In: Shils ME, Shike M, Ross AC, Caballero B, Cousins JR. Modern nutrition in health and disease. 10th edition. Baltimore: Lippincott Williams & Wilkins; 2006. p. 1554-1566.

Sports Performance

Sports Performance

Questions to ask

✓ **Type of sports activity?**

- ○ Intensity? Duration? Frequency? Level of performance?

✓ **Expectations regarding a product in order to improve sports performance?**

✓ **What products have already been used? Other medications taken?**

✓ **Significant medical history?**

- ○ Cardiovascular? Renal? Gastrointestinal?

✓ **Allergies to medications or to foods?**

✓ **Current diet?**

What to do

- Eat a healthy diet: adequate protein, fruit, and vegetable intake

- Following the recommendations of Canada's Food Guide is sufficient for most athletes

- Choose food sources to increase intake of proteins, carbohydrates, and other elements

- Ensure adequate fluid intake: 1 mL/Kcal or 30 mL/kg/day + water losses during physical activity

- Ensure that no product or medication is a substance banned by the Canadian Centre for Ethics in Sport (depending on the desired level of sports performance)

Table I: Breakdown of Energy Intake by Food Source for an Athlete	
Proteins	10%–15%
Fats	< 30%
Carbohydrates (endurance athletes)	60%–70%
Carbohydrates (recreational athletes)	55%–65%

- **Protein intake**
  - Adequate intake is necessary for synthesis of muscular tissue after endurance or resistance exercise. Proteins can also serve as a source of energy
  - Daily recommended intake may vary depending on the level and type of physical exercise

Table II: Daily Recommended Protein Intake (g/kg)	
Basic intake	0.8
Athletes (endurance)	1.2–1.4
Athletes (resistance)	1.6–1.7
Maximum intake	2.0

  - To increase the protein intake without increasing fat intake: use low-fat dairy products, egg whites, chicken, turkey, fish, lean beef, and lean pork
  - Excess protein does not lead to a higher anabolizing effect; the surplus is used in the production of energy
  - Adequate intake of carbohydrates helps to decrease protein utilization during an aerobic endurance activity and thus to maintain a better protein status

- **Carbohydrate intake**
  - A diet rich in carbohydrates helps to maximize muscular and hepatic glycogen reserves before a performance and promotes more rapid replacement of reserves
  - Complex carbohydrates provide a more sustained release of energy

Table III: Suggested Carbohydrate Intake	
Before intense training or competition	1–4.5 g/kg, 1–4 hours before
During exercise or competition	30–60 g/hour
After intense exercise or competition	1–1.5 g/kg in the 30 minutes after, then every 2 hours (take 7–9 g/kg for the 24 hours following the activity)

- o A high dose of carbohydrates (60–70% of calories) during the week before a competition, combined with a decrease in intensity and the duration of exercise, allows for doubling muscular glycogen reserves

- o Recommended for athletes whose competitions last 90 minutes or longer. However, for each gram of glycogen stored, the body stores 2.7 grams of water

What to use

- **Sports drinks**
  - o Contain water and/or electrolytes and/or carbohydrates
  - o More effective than water alone to limit dehydration and increase body temperature during an endurance sports activity
  - o Water (for rehydration): ↓ psychological stress during exercise when it is hot, limits ↑ in body temperature, delays fatigue and improves endurance performance
  - o Electrolytes (sodium): ↑ water absorption, ↓ risk of hyponatremia during an endurance sports activity lasting 4 hours or longer. Replacement of electrolytes is important during a shorter activity (1–2 hours) if it takes place in hot and humid temperatures, especially for athletes who sweat a lot. A salty snack or meal is sufficient for an activity of less than one hour
  - o Carbohydrates: ↑ efficacy for delaying the onset of fatigue. Beneficial for activities of one hour or longer to replace muscular glycogen. Do not affect gastrointestinal tolerance

- Proteins: additional source of energy. Unstable once the powder dissolves in water (to be used within 2 hours). Releases gas during reconstitution, which may influence gastrointestinal tolerance and adversely affect athletes who are not used to it
- Caffeine: ↑ absorption of glucose
- Glycerol: water retention → hyperhydration. Improves cardiovascular response, regulation of temperature, and performance in cycling. No significant advantage in relation to rehydration. Weight gain not desirable for some activities like running
- Noncarbonated beverages are preferred to limit gastrointestinal discomfort. Taking oxygenated water does not affect sports performance

Table I: Characteristics of Various Products

Product	Dosage	Description/Efficacy	Comments
Creatine	Loading dose: 20 g/day or 0.3 g/kg/day (4 doses) x 5 days Maintenance dose: 3–5 g/day or 0.03 g/kg/day	Located in the skeletal muscle in the form of free creatine or high-energy phosphorylated creatine Synthesized by the body or absorbed through food (red meat and fish) Increases muscular performance for short periods of high-intensity exercise Increases muscular strength by approximately 1% per week during resistance training Endurance activity: no beneficial effect for high-intensity activities longer than 20–30 seconds or for other sports performance Muscular concentrations of creatine quickly return to their initial level when administration stops. There is no proof that gains obtained are maintained after the person stops taking creatine Initial weight gain includes a portion of water	Adverse Effects Muscle cramps, dehydration, weight gain, hepatic and renal dysfunction. Gastrointestinal intolerance (divide the loading dose in four). Use seems safe for 5 years and does not seem to affect renal function in healthy athletes Drug interactions Potentially nephrotoxic agents (NSAIDs, ACEIs, cyclosporine), caffeine (may decrease efficacy of creatine) Precautions/contraindications Renal failure or diseases that increase the risk of renal failure, such as diabetes

Table I: Characteristics of Various Products (cont'd)

Product	Dosage	Description/Efficacy	Comments
Protein	Recommended Daily Intake: Resistance: 1.6–1.7 g/kg/day Endurance: 1.2–1.4 g/kg/day	Recommended to increase muscle mass, to prevent protein catabolism during prolonged exercise, to support the synthesis of hemoglobin, myoglobin, and oxidative enzymes during aerobic training and to replace protein lost in sweat and urine during exercise No effect on strength, power, or muscle hypertrophy in athletes who have an adequate dietary protein intake	Adverse Effects Increase in diuresis (excretion of excess nitrogenous wastes) and risk of dehydration if consumed in excess Precautions/contraindications Renal failure (risk of progression of the disease) and osteoporosis (increased excretion of calcium)
Hydroxy-methyl-butyrate (HMB)	1.5–3 g/day (1–3 doses)	Leucine metabolite Mechanism of action is unknown Resistance activity: increase in lean body mass and muscular strength in the elderly, among others. The effect is less pronounced in people who already do resistance training Endurance activity: benefits remain to be proven	Adverse Effects None reported Drug interactions None reported Precautions/contraindications None reported

Table I: Characteristics of Various Products (cont'd)

Product	Dosage	Description/Efficacy	Comments
Chromium picolinate	200–400 µg/day (use the trivalent form only)	Insulin cofactor Mechanism of action: promotes uptake of glucose and amino acids into muscle cells Resistance activity: controversial effect on lean body mass and muscle strength Endurance activity: no effect	Adverse Effects Cognitive, perceptual, and motor dysfunction (200–400 µg/day), anemia, thrombocytopenia, hemolysis, hepatic dysfunction and renal failure (1.2–2.4 mg/day) Picolinic acid affects cerebral metabolism of dopamine, serotonin, and noradrenalin Drug interactions Vitamin C (increase in chromium absorption), insulin (↑ risk of hypoglycemia)
Sodium phosphate	0.3 g/kg/day x 6 days	Buffering effect on lactic acid in the muscles Anaerobic endurance activity: contradictory data, but seems to improve performance (delays the onset of fatigue and increases physical power)	Adverse Effects cramps, nausea, diarrhea in high doses Precautions/contraindications Renal failure
Sodium citrate	0.5 g/kg/day x 6 days	Aerobic endurance activity: possible beneficial effect, but more studies are required	

Table I: Characteristics of Various Products (cont'd)

Product	Dosage	Description/Efficacy	Comments
Caffeine	2–10 mg/kg	Adenosine receptor antagonist and central nervous system stimulant Mechanism of action: unknown, increase in muscle contraction strength versus decrease in psychological perception of the effort Resistance activity: no efficacy Endurance activity: improves performance in aerobic endurance If consumed in moderation, does not create an electrolytic imbalance despite a diuretic effect	<u>Adverse Effects</u> Insomnia, nervousness, akathisia, gastric irritation, nausea, vomiting, tachycardia, tremors, delirium, convulsions, diuresis, withdrawal syndrome (headache, irritability, nervousness, anxiety, dizziness), tolerance, psychological dependence, tachyarrhythmia, and sleep disturbance (250–300 mg/day), severe toxicity leading to death (3–10 g) <u>Drug interactions</u> Creatine (possible → creatine effect), clozapine, central nervous system stimulants, ephedrine, lithium, monoamine oxidase inhibitors (MAOIs), theophylline <u>Precautions/contraindications</u> Gastrointestinal ulcer, cardiac conduction abnormalities, depression, anxiety disorder, diabetes, renal disease, hypertension

- **Other products studied:**
  - Dehydroepiandrosterone (DHEA)
    - Studies on humans show no increase in seric testosterone, but show an increase in seric estradiol and estrone in men (conversion of DHEA by aromatase)
    - Risk of resistance to insulin, of hepatic damage, and of cancer (breast, endometrium, and prostate)
  - L-carnitine
    - No study has shown any ergogenic effect associated with taking L-carnitine supplements to improve aerobic and anaerobic performance. Has shown no effect on decreasing body fat
    - Essential cofactor for carrying long-chain fatty acids into the mitochondria. Synthesized in the liver from lysine and methionine
    - Administration of 5 g of carnitine a day has shown no improvement in VO_2. The putative mechanism is an improved oxidation of lipids and absorption of oxygen
  - Ginseng
    - No effect on athletic performance nor in the delay of onset of fatigue
  - Antioxidants
    - No proof that using antioxidants (carotinoids, glutathion, N-acethylcysteine, coenzyme Q10, Vitamin E, Vitamin C, etc.) reduces oxidative stress during exercise nor the recovery period after exercise
  - Pseudoephedrine
    - No proof that pseudoephedrine in OTC doses improves sports performances
    - This substance is banned in high-level sports
  - Arginine, lysine, and ornithine
    - In high doses, result in transitory increase in concentrations of human growth hormone; this increase is not sufficiently sustained to increase muscle mass or decrease body fat

- ○ Branched-chain amino acids (leucine, isoleucine, and valine)
  - – These amino acids compete with tryptophan (the precursor to serotonin) for brain penetration. They thus delay fatigue in the central nervous system and improve performance during long aerobic endurance activities
  - – Data are contradictory with regard to benefits

References

- Bergeron MF, Waller JL, Marinik EL. Volontary fluid intake and core temperature responses in adolescent tennis players: sport beverage versus water. Br Sports Med. 2006; 40: 406-10.
- Heschuk S. Sports nutrition. In: Repchinsky C, Leblanc C, editors. Patient self-care: helping patients make therapeutic choices. 1st edition. Ottawa: Canadian Pharmacists Association; Welcom Ltd: 2002. p. 397-46.
- Kreider RB, Ferreira M, Wilson M, Grindstaff P, Plisk S, Reinardy J, et al. Effects of creatine supplementation on body composition, strength, and sprint performance. Med Sci Sports Exerc.1998; 30: 73-82.
- Lukaski HC. Magnesium, zinc, and chromium nutriture and physical activity. Am J Clin Nutr. 2000; 72: 585-93.
- Newnham M. Sports nutrition and performance-enhancing nutrients. In: Berardi RR, Kroon LA, McDermott JH, Newton GD, Oszko MA, Popovich NG, et al, editors. Handbook of nonprescription drugs: an interactive approach to self-care. 15th edition. Washington: American Pharmacists Association; 2006. p. 503-20.
- Nissen SL, Sharp RL. Effect of dietary supplements on lean mass and strength gains with resistance exercise: a meta-analysis. J Appl Physiol. 2003; 94: 651-6.
- Peyrebrune MC, Stokes K, Hall GM, Nevill ME. Effect of creatine supplementation on training for competition in elite swimmers. Med Sci Sports Exerc. 2005; 37:2140-7.
- Poortmans JR, Francaux M. Long-term oral creatine supplementation doest not impair renal function in healthy athletes. Med Sci Sports Exerc. 1999; 31:1108-10.
- Williams MH. Sports nutrition. In: Shils ME, Shike M, Ross AC, Caballero B, Cousins JR. Modern nutrition in health and disease. 10th edition. Baltimore: Lippincott Williams & Wilkins; 2006. p. 1723-1739.
- Van Nieuwenhoven MA, Brummer R-JM, Brouns F. Gastrointestinal function during exercise: comparison of water, sports drink, and sports drink with caffeine. J Appl Physiol. 2000; 89. p. 1079-85.

Natural Products

Natural Products

Questions to ask

- ✓ Why the need for a natural product?
- ✓ What are the symptoms?
- ✓ What is the patient's medical history?
- ✓ Other medications taken?
- ✓ Other natural products taken?
- ✓ Natural products or medications already tried?
- ✓ Pregnancy or breastfeeding?
- ✓ Diagnosed health problems or illnesses?
- ✓ Presence of allergies to medications, foods, or plants?
- ✓ Preferred product brand?

What to use

- Information on natural products is not exhaustive and is based on the available documentation. Consequently, these products should be recommended and used with diligence

- The products dealt with in this chapter are presented by system in the following order:

  - Cardiovascular System
    - Hypercholesterolemia: beta-sitosterol, blond psyllium, garlic, flaxseed, fish oil
    - Hypertension: garlic, fish oil

  - Gastrointestinal Tract
    - Constipation: cascara, blond psyllium, flaxseed, senna
    - Dyspepsia: artichoke, calcium
    - Nausea: ginger, pyridoxine

o <u>Urogenital Tract</u>
  - Erectile dysfunction: L-arginine
  - Benign prostatic hyperplasia: beta-sitosterol, African plum, saw palmetto, red clover
  - Urinary infection (prophylaxis): cranberry

o <u>Immune System</u>
  - Labial herpes: lemon balm, lysine
  - Cold/common flu: echinacea, zinc (lozenge), Vitamin C

o <u>Musculoskeletal System</u>
  - Degenerative joint disease (osteoarthritis): chondroitin, glucosamine, S-adenosylmethionine (SAMe), capsaicin
  - Fibromyalgia: magnesium and malic acid, SAMe,

o <u>Central Nervous System</u>
  - Anxiety: St. John's Wort, passionflower, valerian
  - Depression: St. John's Wort, SAMe, EPA
  - Insomnia: valerian, passionflower, melatonin

o <u>Women's Health</u>
  - Menopause: black cohosh, flaxseed, soy, red clover
  - Premenstrual syndrome: chasteberry, magnesium, ginkgo biloba
  - Premenstrual dysphoric disorder: chasteberry

Cardiovascular System					
Product	Dosage	Adverse Effects	Precautions	Interactions	Comments
Hypercholesterolemia					
Beta-sitosterol	0.8–6 g/day before meals (divided doses)	Nausea, diarrhea, constipation, indigestion, flatulence Possible erectile dysfunction and ↓ libido	Pregnancy and breastfeeding: little data, to be avoided Sitosterolemia (contraindicated)	Carotenes and Vitamin E (↓ their absorption) Ezetimibe (↓ absorption of beta-sitosterol)	↓ absorption of cholesterol due to competition (↓ in total cholesterol and in LDL cholesterol, no effect on HDL cholesterol) Data available up to 18 months of use
Blond psyllium (*Plantago ovata*)	Ground husks: 3.4 g po tid or 5.1 g po bid Whole seeds can also be used. Do not chew, crush, or grind seeds (nephrotoxic pigment)	Flatulence, abdominal pain, dyspepsia, diarrhea (transitory: start with a smaller dose), constipation, esophageal and intestinal obstruction (if insufficient water intake), headache, back pain, rhinitis, allergic reaction which can progress to anaphylaxis	Pregnancy and breastfeeding: safe Dysphagia, obstructive gastrointestinal disorders Prior allergic reaction	<u>Pharmacodynamic:</u> Insulin and oral hypoglycemic agents (hypoglycemic effect) <u>Pharmacokinetic:</u> Vitamins and minerals (iron, lithium, etc.), carbamazepine, digoxin, warfarin, and other po medications (↓ absorption)	4% ↓ in total cholesterol and 7% ↓ in LDL cholesterol compared with the placebo (combined with a reduced-fat diet). No effect on triglycerides or on HDL cholesterol ↑ efficacy of simvastatin Drink plenty of water (240 mL per 3.5–5.1 g of husks or 7 g of seeds)

Cardiovascular System (cont'd)					
Product	Dosage	Adverse Effects	Precautions	Interactions	Comments
Hypercholesterolemia (cont'd)					
Garlic (*Allium sativum*)	Fresh: 4 g (~ 1 clove/day (alliin 1%) Extract: 600– 1200 mg/day (divided into three doses) (standardized extract: alliin 1.3%)	Garlic breath and body odour, mouth and gastrointestinal irritation, flatulence, nausea, vomiting, diarrhea, belching, sweating, weakness, sense of inebriation, alteration of the gastrointestinal flora, bleeding	Pregnancy (abortive in high doses) and breastfeeding (avoid high doses, changes taste of the milk) Coagulation disorders (stop taking 7–10 days before surgery), gastrointestinal irritation (caution during infection or gastrointestinal inflammation)	Induces the isoenzyme CYP2E1, 3A4 Pharmacodynamic: anticoagulants, antiplatelet drugs (↑ INR), oral hypoglycemic agents, insulin, antihypertensives Pharmacokinetic: oral contraceptives, cyclosporine (↓ efficacy), isoniazid, NNRTI, saquinavir (major)	Contradictory data A slight decrease in LDL was observed, but the effect is not sustained Data available up to 4 years of use
Flaxseed (*Linum usitatissimum*)	40–50 g po/day (ground seeds)	Bloating, flatulence, abdominal pain, diarrhea, constipation, dyspepsia, nausea, intestinal obstruction (if insufficient water intake), allergic reaction	Pregnancy and breastfeeding: little data, to be avoided Coagulation disorders, gastrointestinal obstruction (to be avoided) cancer of the breast, uterus, and ovaries endometriosis, uterine fibroids, known allergy	Pharmacodynamic: anticoagulants, increases action of antiplatelet drugs, increases action of hypoglycemic agents and insulin Pharmacokinetic: ↓ absorption of other medications	Take with water (150 mL per 15 mL of ground seeds) ↓ total cholesterol and LDL cholesterol in the presence of hypercholesterolemia and of normal cholesterolemia

Cardiovascular System (cont'd)

Product	Dosage	Adverse Effects	Precautions	Interactions	Comments
Hypercholesterolemia (cont'd)					
Fish oil (source of omega-3 fatty acids)	1–4 g po/day	Fish taste, halitosis, belching, epistaxis, nausea, pyrosis, soft stools, fecal incontinence, rash, bleeding (> 9 g/day), ↓ immune function, vitamin (A and D) toxicity, mercury toxicity	Pregnancy and breastfeeding: Little data, beware of mercury Diabetes (↑ postprandial glycemia), cirrhosis (↑ risk of bleeding) Hypersensitivity to ASA (↓ pulmonary function), bipolar disease (risk of hypomania), decreased immunity (↓ immune and inflammatory response), allergy to seafood	Pharmacodynamic: anticoagulants, antiplatelet drugs (↓ platelet aggregation), antihypertensives (additive effect) Pharmacokinetic: Orlistat (↓ fat absorption)	20–50% ↓ in triglycerides Could possibly improve the fat profile
Hypertension					
Garlic Ail (*Allium sativum*)	See "Hyper-cholesterolemia"	See "Hyper-cholesterolemia"	See "Hyper-cholesterolemia"	See "Hyper-cholesterolemia"	Efficacy not demonstrated for hypertension Modest decrease in blood pressure of 2–7% after 4 weeks Data available up to 4 years of use

Cardiovascular System (cont'd)

Product	Dosage	Adverse Effects	Precautions	Interactions	Comments
Hypertension (cont'd)					
Fish oil (source of omega-3 fatty acids)	4 g po/day	See "Hyper-cholesterolemia"	See "Hyper-cholesterolemia"	See "Hyper-cholesterolemia"	Modest ↓ in systolic and diastolic blood pressure in mild hypertensive patients
Blond psyllium (*Plantago ovata*)	Ground husks: 15 g po/day	See "Hyper-cholesterolemia"	See "Hyper-cholesterolemia"	See "Hyper-cholesterolemia"	Seems to ↓ diastolic blood pressure and systolic blood pressure when taken with soy protein Take with plenty of water (240 mL per 3.5–5.1 g of husks or 7 g of seeds)

Gastrointestinal Tract

Product	Dosage	Adverse Effects	Precautions	Interactions	Comments
Constipation					
Cascara (*Frangula purshiana*)	20–30 mg po/day (cascaroside A) 2 g of bark in infusion 2–5 mL po tid (liquid extract)	Discomfort and abdominal cramps, diarrhea, colouring of urine and mucosa Chronic use (> 1–2 weeks): hypokalemia, dependency, colitis, muscular weakness, cachexia	Pregnancy (insufficient data) and breastfeeding (diarrhea possible) Intestinal obstruction, irritable bowel syndrome, inflammatory bowel diseases, abdominal pain of unknown etiology, ulceration	<u>Pharmacodynamic:</u> Digoxin (contains glycosides) Corticosteroids, diuretics and other laxatives (↑ risk of hypokalemia) <u>Pharmacokinetic:</u> ↓ absorption of other medications (↓ GI transit)	Stimulating laxative Limit use to 1–2 weeks

Gastrointestinal Tract (cont'd)					
Product	Dosage	Adverse Effects	Precautions	Interactions	Comments
Constipation (cont'd)					
Blond psyllium (*Plantago ovata*)	Seeds: 7–40 g/day (divided doses bid–qid) after meals Do not chew, crush, or grind seeds (nephrotoxic pigment)	See "Hyper-cholesterolemia"	See "Hyper-cholesterolemia"	See "Hyper-cholesterolemia"	Laxative through mass effect and fecal emollient Drink plenty of water (240 mL per 3.5–5.1 g of husks or 7 g of seeds)
Flaxseed (*Linum usitatissimum*)	15 mL po bid–tid (ground seeds)	See "Hyper-cholesterolemia"	See "Hyper-cholesterolemia"	See "Hyper-cholesterolemia"	Laxative through mass effect Take with water (150 mL per 15 mL ground seeds)
Senna (*Senna alexandria*)	15–30 mg po/day (sennoside B) 0.5–2 g dried leaves in infusion bid prn, soaking the dried leaves in cold water for 10–12 h	See "Cascara" Damage to colonic musculature The cold tea causes fewer GI effects	See "Cascara" Pregnancy and breastfeeding: to be avoided	<u>Pharmacodynamic:</u> Corticosteroids, diuretics, and other laxatives (↑ risk of hypokalemia)	Do not use in boiling water

		Gastrointestinal Tract (cont'd)			
Product	Dosage	Adverse Effects	Precautions	Interactions	Comments
Dyspepsia					
Artichoke (*Cynara scolymus*)	320–640 mg qd (leaf extract 12:1) 2 g dried leaves tid	Flatulence, contact dermatitis, allergic reaction	Pregnancy and breastfeeding: little data Allergy to chrysanthemums obstruction of bile ducts, stones		Onset of action: 2–6 weeks
Nausea					
Ginger (*Zingiber officinale*)	**Motion sickness:** 1 g dry powder 30 min before departure and q4h prn **Nausea:** 0.25–1 g po tid (dried root) or as an infusion Maximum 4 g/day *Gravol* natural source (500 mg of ginger root per tablet): 2 tablets every 4 h prn, maximum 6 tablets/day	Dermatitis, diarrhea, dyspepsia, irritation of mucosa, depression of central nervous system and arrhythmia if overdose	Pregnancy and breastfeeding: insufficient data at high doses Kidney stones, bleeding, heart disease, coagulopathies, diabetes	Pharmacodynamic: Anticoagulants, antiplatelet drugs antihypertensives (↑ and ↓ blood pressure) PPI, H₂-receptor antagonist and antacids (↑ gastric acidity), CNS depressants, insulin and oral hypoglycemic agents (↓ glycemia), barbiturates and heart medications (inotropic effect)	More effective than a placebo and equivalent to pyridoxine in treating nausea during pregnancy Prevention of post-op nausea and vomiting (ginger not effective in the presence of narcotic anesthesia or analgesia)

Gastrointestinal Tract (cont'd)

Product	Dosage	Adverse Effects	Precautions	Interactions	Comments
Nausea (cont'd)					
Vitamin B$_6$ Pyridoxine	10–25 mg po tid (doses used in pregnancy)	Nausea, vomiting, abdominal pain, ↓ appetite, headache, paresthesia, ↑ AST, ↓ folic acid, drowsiness, cutaneous reaction, allergic reaction	Angioplasty: may ↑ the risk of restenosis in combination with Vitamin B$_{12}$ and folic acid	Pharmacodynamic: Amiodarone (photosensitivity) Pharmacokinetic: Levodopa (↑ peripheral metabolism if no carbidopa), phenytoin, phenobarbital (↓ concentration)	Studies carried out on pregnant women

Urogenital Tract

Product	Dosage	Adverse Effects	Precautions	Interactions	Comments
Erectile Dysfunction					
L-arginine	5 g po qd	Abdominal pain, nausea, diarrhea, bloating, gout, allergic reaction, metabolic acidosis and hyperkalemia possible at high doses. Well tolerated ad 30 g/day	Pregnancy and breastfeeding: insufficient data Asthma, (allergic exacerbation), hypotension, liver cirrhosis, renal failure, herpes simplex type II, hyperuricemia, sickle cell anemia	Pharmacodynamic: Antihypertensives, nitrates, PDE–5 inhibitors ACEIs, diuretics saving K$^+$	Substrate in the production of nitric oxide which has a vasodilating effect Subjective improvement when organic erectile dysfunction Taking 9 g per day for 6 months seems well tolerated

Urogenital Tract (cont'd)					
Product	Dosage	Adverse Effects	Precautions	Interactions	Comments
Benign Prostatic Hyperplasia					
Beta-sitosterol	60–130 mg po/day divided bid–tid	See "Hyper-cholesterolemia"	See "Hyper-cholesterolemia"	See "Hyper-cholesterolemia"	Inhibition of 5-α-reductase Improvement of symptoms and urinary flow, ↓ residual urinary volume, no effect on the size of the prostate Data available ad 18 months of use
African Plum (*Prunus africana*)	50–100 mg po bid (standardized lipophilic extract: 14% triterpenes, 0.5% n-docosanol)	Nausea, diarrhea, constipation, pyrosis		None known	Improvement in urinary flow, residual urinary volume, urinary frequency, and subjective symptoms
Saw palmetto (*Srenoa repens*)	1–2 g (whole fruit) 160 mg po bid or 320 mg po qd (lipophilic extract: ~85% fatty acids)	Headache, nausea, vomiting, diarrhea, possible erectile dysfunction		Hormonal therapy	Seems to inhibit 5-α-reductase Slightly to moderately improves symptoms and urinary flow Onset of action: 2 months Seems safe ad 48 weeks

	Urogenital Tract (cont'd)				
Product	Dosage	Adverse Effects	Precautions	Interactions	Comments
Benign Prostatic Hyperplasia (cont'd)					
Red clover (Trifolium pratense) Source of isoflavone	4 g of flower po tid (whole or as infusion)	Rash	Coagulation disorders, estrogen-sensitive conditions	Hormonal therapies (estrogen, progesterone), coumarin anticoagulants, antiplatelet drugs	↓ frequency of nocturia, improvement in symptoms and in quality of life In Australia, Trinivin is marketed for benign prostatic hyperplasia
Urinary Infections (prophylaxis)					
Cranberry (Vaccinium macrocarpon)	Juice cocktail: 90 mL po/day Fresh or frozen fruit: 30 g 1.5 g of fresh fruit = 1 L of juice Juice cocktail: pure juice (3:1)	Diarrhea, gastrointestinal symptoms (3–4 L/day)	Diabetes (sweetened juice)	CYP2C9 inhibitor Pharmacokinetic: Warfarin Pharmacodynamic: PPI	Seems to decrease the frequency of urinary tract infections in women and in elderly women Helps combat bad odour in incontinent patients

	Immune System				
Product	Dosage	Adverse Effects	Precautions	Interactions	Comments
Herpes labialis					
Lemon Balm (*Melissa officinalis*)	Cream or ointment 1% (70:1 aqueous lyophilized extract) applied locally bid-qid from appearance of prodromal signs ad healing (max. 14 days) Infusion: 2–3 tablespoons of ground leaves in 150 mL boiling water, applied locally with a cotton swab	Skin irritation, hypersensitivity reaction	Pregnancy and breastfeeding: insufficient data		Can decrease the intensity and duration of symptoms, as well as the number and size of lesions Does not reduce the risk of transmission Chronic application may reduce the frequency of recurrence
Lysine	1000 mg po qd x 12 months or 1000 mg po tid x 6 months	Diarrhea, abdominal pain (at high doses)	Pregnancy and breastfeeding: insufficient data Kidney disease (one case of tubulointerstitial nephritis)	<u>Pharmacokinetic:</u> Calcium (↑ absorption and ↓ renal excretion of Ca^{2+})	Reduces the frequency of recurrence, its severity, and healing time Data available ad 18 months of use at 1000 mg/day

Immune System (cont'd)

Product	Dosage	Adverse Effects	Precautions	Interactions	Comments
Cold/Flu					
Echinacea (*Echinacea purpurea, angustifolia, pallida*)	2 tablets po tid (6.78 mg/tablet extract of echinacea purpurea) Juice: 6–9 mL po qd	Nausea, vomiting, diarrhea, fever, allergic reaction (anaphylaxis, asthma, urticaria, angioedema), tingling of the tongue	Pregnancy and breastfeeding Autoimmune diseases or immunity disorders, known allergy to chrysanthemums, atopy (↑ risk of allergic reaction), diabetes (↓ metabolic control—parenterally), fertility problems	CYP3A4 inhibitor No interaction reported in humans Pharmacodynamic: Immunosuppressors (↓ efficacy)	Slightly reduces the severity and duration of flu symptoms in adults when taken upon appearance of symptoms, but data are controversial Long-term use can adversely impact the immune system (limit daily use to 8 weeks)
Zinc (lozenges)	1 lozenge every 2 waking hours upon appearance of symptoms (let melt in the mouth) (Zn²⁺/lozenge: 13.3–23 mg) Content Zn²⁺ ZnSO₄ 22.7% Zinc gluconate: 14.3%	Metallic taste, nausea, vomiting, diarrhea, irritation and mucosal erosion of gastrointestinal tract, tubular necrosis, interstitial nephritis	Pregnancy (safe ad 25 mg/day) and breastfeeding (daily recommended value: 16–19 mg/day) HIV (avoid high doses; ↓ survival), hemochromatosis (use with caution)	Pharmacodynamic: Cisplatin (↑ cytoxicity of cisplatin if taken with EDTA) Pharmacokinetic: Coffee (50% ↓ absorption of Zn²⁺), fluoroquinolones, tetracyclines (↓ absorption), K+ sparing diuretics, thiazide-like diuretics, captopril	↓ duration of symptoms in adults and children

Immune System (cont'd)

Cold/Flu (cont'd)

Product	Dosage	Adverse Effects	Precautions	Interactions	Comments
Vitamin C (ascorbic acid)	Treatment: 1–3 g po qd Prevention during physical stress: 0.6–1 g qd Take 2 hours after meal	Depending on the dose: nausea, vomiting, diarrhea, esophagitis, pyrosis, abdominal cramps, gastrointestinal obstruction, vasomotor flushing, headache, insomnia, drowsiness At high doses: osmotic diarrhea (> 2 g/day), nephrolithiasis, deep vein thrombosis, possible scurvy upon stopping	Pregnancy (avoid high doses) and breastfeeding (max. 1.8–2.0 g/day) Diabetes (↑ glycemia possible), G6PD deficiency, nephrolithiasis (> 1 g/day: 40% ↑ risk), iron overload, sickle cell anemia, hemochromatosis, thalassemia, sideroblastic anemia (use with caution) Diabetic postmenopausal woman (max. 300 mg/day) Angioplasty (avoid before and after)	Pharmacodynamic: Chemotherapy (possible ↓ efficacy through antioxidation effect), statin, niacin (may cause ↑ in HDL cholesterol) Pharmacokinetic: Aluminum, copper, iron, and chromium (↑ their absorption), indinavir (14% ↓ indinavir concentration), warfarin (possible ↓ absorption)	Contradictory data Assess risks vs benefits (↑ risk of adverse effects at recommended doses)

Musculoskeletal System

Degenerative Joint Disease (Osteoarthritis)

Product	Dosage	Adverse Effects	Precautions	Interactions	Comments
Chondroitin (sulfate)	200–400 mg bid-tid or 1200 mg po/day in a single dose or take intermittently: 800 mg po/day for 3 months, stop 3 months then resume	Well tolerated Nausea, epigastric pain, diarrhea, constipation, eyelid edema, edema of lower limbs, headache, alopecia, extrasystoles, allergic reaction, possible anticoagulant effect	Pregnancy and breastfeeding: insufficient data Coagulopathy, renal failure (↑ t½), asthma, (exacerbation possible) prostate cancer (avoid: ↑ possible spreading and recurrence)	Pharmacodynamic: Anticoagulants (↑ INR and anti-Xa activity possible), antiplatelet drugs	Present in joint cartilage Contradictory data Could ↓ pain and progression Low bioavailability (0–13%) Topical application: insufficient data Data available ad 6 months of use Long-term safety: insufficient data
Glucosamine (sulfate)	1500 mg po/day (dose separated qd–tid) Take with food	Nausea, pyrosis, diarrhea, constipation drowsiness, cutaneous reaction, headache, ↑ glycemia (controversial)	Pregnancy and breastfeeding Asthma, (exacerbation possible), diabetes (↑ glycemia), hypertension (possible ↑ blood pressure), allergy to crustaceans (cross-allergy unlikely)	Pharmacodynamic: Anticoagulants, antiplatelet drugs (↑ INR), oral hypoglycemic agents, insulin, Etoposide, teniposide, doxorubicin (↓ topoisomerase II inhibitor)	Plays a role in cartilage synthesis Decreases pain, improves mobility and ↓ progression at the knee level After 8 weeks, seems more effective than ibuprofen at 1.2 g/day Improvement in 4–8 weeks Topical application: insufficient data Data available ad 3 years of use

Musculoskeletal System (cont'd)

Degenerative Joint Disease (Osteoarthritis) (cont'd)

Product	Dosage	Adverse Effects	Precautions	Interactions	Comments
SAMe (S-adenosyl-L-methionine)	200 mg po tid	Flatulence, nausea, vomiting, diarrhea, headache (depending on the dose) Anxiety, hypomania, mania	Pregnancy (possibly safe in the 3rd trimester, but insufficient data) and breastfeeding (insufficient data) Bipolar disease (hypomania, mania), depression (↑ anxiety)	Pharmacodynamic: Antidepressants (5-HT additive effects)	Efficacy (> placebo and ~ NSAIDs) for ↓ symptoms Onset of action: 30 days (vs 15 days with NSAIDs) Data available ad 2 years of use
Capsicum (Capsicum sp.)	Cream (0.025% –0.075%) local topical application tid–qid x 4 weeks	Burning sensation, erythema, irritation (↓ with prolonged use), urticaria Very irritating for eyes and mucous membranes	Pregnancy and breastfeeding: safe in topical application Wounds (do not apply directly), pepper allergy (avoid)	Pharmacodynamic: ACEIs (exacerbation of cough reflex), anticoagulants, antiplatelet drugs	Temporary relief from pain Onset of action: 3 days, but may take ad 14 days for the complete analgesic effect Clean with diluted vinegar (lipophilic, cannot be cleaned with water alone) Wash hands after application

Musculoskeletal System (cont'd)

Product	Dosage	Adverse Effects	Precautions	Interactions	Comments
Fibromyalgia					
Magnesium and malic acid	4–6 tablets po bid (*SuperMalic*) (Mg(OH)$_2$ 200–300 mg + malic acid 800–1200 mg bid)	Gastrointestinal irritation, nausea, vomiting, diarrhea	Pregnancy and breastfeeding: insufficient data Heart blockage (avoid), renal failure (hypermagnesemia)	<u>Pharmacodynamic</u>: Muscle relaxants <u>Pharmacokinetic</u>: Quinolones, biphosphonates, tetracyclines (↓ absorption)	↓ in pain and sensitivity
SAMe (S-adenosyl-L-methionine)	800 mg po/day	See "Degenerative Joint Disease/ Osteoarthritis"	See "Degenerative Joint Disease/ Osteoarthritis"	See "Degenerative Joint Disease/ Osteoarthritis"	Improvement of symptoms vs placebo Little data available at 2 years of use

| Central Nervous System |||||||
Product	Dosage	Adverse Effects	Precautions	Interactions	Comments
Anxiety						
St. John's Wort (*Hypericum perforatum*)	300–1200 mg po/day (standardized extract: hypericin 0.3%) Do not exceed 1800 mg/day	Insomnia, agitated sleep, anxiety, agitation, irritability, gastrointestinal discomfort, fatigue, dry mouth, dizziness, headache, paresthesia, hypomania, mania, photosensitivity, phototoxicity, withdrawal syndrome, possible sexual dysfunction	Pregnancy (↑ uterine tone) and breastfeeding (adverse effects in infants) Bipolar disease, severe depression, infertility	Induces CYP3A4, 2C9, 2D6, 1A2, and P-gp **Pharmacodynamic:** Antidepressants, 5-HT₁ agonists (triptans), photosensitizing agents **Pharmacokinetic:** Cyclosporine, digoxin, antiretrovirals (NNRTI, PI), oral contraceptives, theophylline, warfarin, olanzapine	Seems safe if used for 8 weeks Some data suggest efficacy in treating anxiety
Passionflower (*Passiflora incarnata*)	0.25–2 g po tid prn (dried plant or as infusion)	Vasculitis, confusion, pancreatic toxicity, withdrawal syndrome	Pregnancy (uterine stimulation) and breastfeeding (insufficient data)	**Pharmacodynamic:** CNS depressants MAOIs (↑ effect of MAOIs)	Studied in combination with other plants Little date on monotherapy

Central Nervous System (cont'd)					
Product	Dosage	Adverse Effects	Precautions	Interactions	Comments
Anxiety (cont'd)					
Valerian (*Valeriana officinalis*)	Variable 50 mg po tid (ad 9/day) or 450 mg po tid (standardized extract: valerianic acid 0.3–0.6%)	Headache, drowsiness, insomnia, excitability, dry mouth, GI irritation, withdrawal syndrome, liver toxicity (long-term, idiosyncratic use)	Pregnancy (uterine contractions) and breastfeeding (insufficient data) Hepatic disorders	CYP3A4 substrates <u>Pharmacodynamic:</u> CNS depressants	Avoid driving or operating heavy machinery Onset of action: 2–4 weeks Improvement in psychic symptoms of HAM-A Improvement in response to laboratory-induced stress ↓ benzodiazepine withdrawal symptoms
Depression					
St. John's Wort (*Hypericum perforatum*)	300 mg po tid (standardized extract: hypericin 0.3%) Do not exceed 1800 mg per day	See "Anxiety"	See "Anxiety"	Induces CYP3A4, 2C9, 2D6, 1A2, and P-gp (See "Anxiety")	See "Anxiety" Contradictory data Modest efficacy (> placebo) as treatment for major depression Efficacy (~ paroxetine) as treatment for moderate to severe depression

Central Nervous System (cont'd)

Product	Dosage	Adverse Effects	Precautions	Interactions	Comments
Depression (cont'd)					
SAMe (S-adenosyl-L-methionine)	400–1600 mg po/day (most studied dose: 1600 mg/day)	See "Degenerative Joint Disease/ Osteoarthritis"	See "Degenerative Joint Disease/ Osteoarthritis"	See "Degenerative Joint Disease/ Osteoarthritis"	Mostly studied parenterally for short-term treatment, where it seems effective Effectiveness > placebo Study required to confirm efficacy of oral administration vs antidepressants Onset of action: 1–2 weeks (IV) Data available ad 2 years of use
EPA (eicosa-pentaenoic acid → omega-3 fatty acid)	1 g po bid (fish oil: EPA + DHA)	Fish taste, belching, epistaxis, nausea, soft stools	Pregnancy and breastfeeding: insufficient data Diabetes (interferes with control of glycemia), hypertension (↓ blood pressure in hypertensive patients), hypersensitivity to acetylsalicylic acid (↓ pulmonary function)	<u>Pharmacodynamic:</u> Anticoagulants, antiplatelet drugs, antihypertensives	Significant improvement of symptoms compared with placebo after 2 weeks of treatment when combined with antidepressant treatment

Central Nervous System (cont'd)					
Product	Dosage	Adverse Effects	Precautions	Interactions	Comments
Insomnia					
Valerian (*Valeriana officinalis*)	400–900 mg po before bedtime (2 hours before) (standardized extract: valerianic acid 0.3–0.6%)	See "Anxiety" Controversial residual morning effect (↓ level of alertness and of concentration, drowsiness) Effect is dose-dependent and is pronounced in the hours following intake	See "Anxiety"	See "Anxiety"	See "Anxiety" Decrease in time to fall asleep and improvement in sleep quality. No effect on total duration of sleep Effect possibly unsustained
Passionflower (*Passiflora incarnata*)	0.25–2 g po tid prn (dried plant or as infusion)	See "Anxiety"	See "Anxiety"	See "Anxiety"	Possible efficacy for light insomnia
Melatonin 5-methoxy-N-acetyltryptamine	Variable 0.3–5 mg po at bedtime	Headache, transitory depression symptoms, diurnal fatigue, drowsiness, dizziness, irritability, abdominal cramps	Pregnancy (possible contraceptive effect at high doses) and breastfeeding (insufficient data) Depression (↑ dysphoria), hepatic disease (metabolized in the liver), convulsive disorders (possible ↑ incidence)	Pharmacodynamic: CNS depressants, immunosuppressors (possible ↓ immunosuppressive effect)	Avoid driving or operating heavy machinery x 4–5 h after taking Data available ad 2 months of use

Women's Health					
Product	Dosage	Adverse Effects	Precautions	Interactions	Comments
Menopause					
Black cohosh (*Actaea racemosa*)	2–4 tablets (40–80 mg) po bid ad 6–12 months (1 mg triterpenes glycosides/tablet 20 mg).	Gastrointestinal irritation, headache, rash, dizziness, weight gain, heaviness in legs, cramps, vaginal bleeding, possible liver toxicity	Pregnancy and breastfeeding Breast cancer, cancer of the uterus/ovaries, fibroids, endometriosis, hepatic disorders, renal transplant (rejection setting), high risk of thrombosis	Weak CYP2D6 inhibitor Pharmacodynamic: Cisplatin (↓ cytotoxic effect) Hepatoxic medications	↓ symptoms (hot flashes) Safe for use ad 6 months. Data available ad 1 year of use Long-term effects on cardiovascular diseases, osteoporosis, and breast cancer unknown
Flaxseed (*Linum usitatissimum*)	40 g ground flaxseed po qd	See "Hyper-cholesterolemia"	See "Hyper-cholesterolemia"	See "Hyper-cholesterolemia"	↓ mild symptoms similar to hormone replacement therapy Take with water (150 mL per 15 mL of ground seeds)

Women's Health (cont'd)

Menopause (cont'd)

Product	Dosage	Adverse Effects	Precautions	Interactions	Comments
Soy (*Glycine max*)	Soy protein: 20–60 g per day (34–76 mg of isoflavones/day) or Isoflavones: 35–100 mg/day Genistein: 54 mg/day	Constipation, diarrhea, nausea, bloating, insomnia, headache (migraines), allergic reaction, cutaneous rash, pruritus (rare)	Pregnancy and breastfeeding; estrogenic effect. Cancer of the breast, uterus, ovaries, or bladder; atopy (↑ risk of allergy), hypothyroidism (exacerbation if low iodine reserve), renal failure, nephrolithiasis (contains oxalate), cow-milk allergy (cross-allergy frequent in children)	Pharmacodynamic: Anticoagulants, antiplatelet drugs (↓ platelet aggregation) Pharmacokinetic: Antibiotics (↓ effect of isoflavones because of a ↓ metabolism of intestinal bacterial flora), hormone replacement therapy (competitive inhibition), tamoxifen (↓ antitumour efficacy)	Maximum effect after 2 months of use Modest ↓ in intensity and frequency of hot flashes
Red clover (*Trifolium pratense*) Source of isoflavones	40–80 mg/day (standardized isoflavones) Avoid higher doses	See "Benign prostatic hyperplasia"	See "Benign prostatic hyperplasia"	See "Benign prostatic hyperplasia"	↓ loss of bone mineral density in the spine of pre- and peri-menopausal women but not in postmenopausal women In Australia, *Promensil* is marketed as estrogen replacement

Women's Health (cont'd)

Product	Dosage	Adverse Effects	Precautions	Interactions	Comments
Premenstrual Syndrome					
Chasteberry (*Vitex agnus-castus*)	Variable doses: 4–20 mg per day (Raw extract, often standardized: agnus 6%)	Generally well tolerated Gastrointestinal disorders, nausea, diarrhea, headache, pruritus, urticaria, rash, acne, insomnia, weight gain, irregular menstrual bleeding	Pregnancy and breastfeeding: hormonal effect, avoid Cancer of the breast, uterus, and ovaries; endometriosis; uterine fibroids; in vitro fertilization (↓ chances of success)	Pharmacodynamic: Dopaminergic agonists and antagonists, hormonal contraceptives, hormone replacement therapy (hormonal effect)	Effect ≥ placebo: ↓ symptoms (mastalgia, edema, constipation, irritability, moods, anger, headache) after three menstrual cycles of treatment Not effective for bloating Data available ad 18 months of use
Magnesium	200–360 mg Mg²⁺/day	Gastrointestinal irritation, nausea, vomiting, diarrhea, hypermagnesemia (thirst, hypotension, drowsiness, confusion, muscular weakness, cardiac arrhythmia, coma, etc.) Doses > 350 mg/day: ↑ risk of diarrhea	Pregnancy and breastfeeding: avoid high doses Renal failure; heart blockage (↑ risk if hypermagnesemia), restless leg syndrome (↑ risk but also treats this disorder)	Pharmacodynamic: Aminoglycosides, muscle relaxants Pharmacokinetic: Calcium, zinc (↓ absorption), Vitamin D (↑ absorption), biphosphonates, quinolones, tetracyclines	Seems to relieve symptoms (mood, water/fluid retention) Seems to prevent premenstrual migraines

Women's Health (cont'd)					
Product	Dosage	Adverse Effects	Precautions	Interactions	Comments
Premenstrual Syndrome (cont'd)					
Ginkgo (*Ginkgo biloba*)	80 mg po bid (from the 16th day of the cycle to the 5th day of the next cycle) (leaf extract) Do not consume fresh ginkgo seeds or more than 10 roasted seeds	GI disorders, headache, drowsiness, palpitations, constipation, cutaneous allergic reaction High dose: akathesia, diarrhea, nausea, vomiting, ↓ muscular tone, weakness, spontaneous bleeding	Pregnancy (induction of labour and hormone effect) and breastfeeding Coagulation disorder (↓ platelet aggregation), type 2 diabetes, perioperative period, epilepsy (neurotoxic ginkgotoxin), infertility (↓ fertility)	Inhibits CYP1A4, 2C9, 2D6, 3A4 Induces CYP2C19, 3A4 Pharmacodynamic: Anticoagulants, antiplatelet drugs, anticonvulsants, products ↓ convulsive threshold, oral hypoglycemic agents, insulin Pharmacokinetic: Alprazolam (↓ absorption)	Relieves mastalgia and neuropsychological symptoms Stop taking 2 weeks before an operation (antiplatelet effect) Data available ad 1 year of use

Women's Health (cont'd)					
Product	Dosage	Adverse Effects	Precautions	Interactions	Comments
Premenstrual Dysphoric Disorder					
Chasteberry (*Vitex agnus-castus*)	Variable doses: 20–240 mg/day in 2–3 divided doses (max 1800 mg/day) Raw extract, often standardized: agnus 6%)	See "Premenstrual Syndrome"	See "Premenstrual Syndrome"	See "Premenstrual Syndrome"	Efficacy comparable to fluoxetine: > fluoxetine: physical symptoms (mastalgia, swelling, cramps, excessive need to eat) < fluoxetine: psychological symptoms (depression, irritability, insomnia, nervousness, sense of losing control) Data available ad 18 months of use

References

- Anderson JW, Allgood LD, Lawrence A, Altringer LA, Jerdack GR, Hengehold DA. Cholesterol-lowering effects of psyllium intake adjunctive to diet therapy in men and women with hypercholesterolemia: meta-analysis of 8 controlled trials. Am J Clin Nutr. 2000; 71:472-9.

- Attele AS, Xie, J-T, Yuan C-S. Treatment of insomnia: an alternative approach. Alternative Medicine Review 2000; 5:249-59.

- Facts and Comparisons. Complementary therapy. In: Nonprescription drug therapy: guiding patient self-care. 5th edition. St-Louis: Facts and Comparisons; 2006. p. 911-1008.

- Hadley S, Petry JJ. Valerian. AM Fam Physician. 2003; 67:1755-8.

- Jellin JM, Gregory PJ, Batz F, Hitchens K, et al. Pharmacist's letter/Prescriber's letter natural medicines comprehensive database. 7th edition. [Internet]. Stockton CA: Therapeutic Research Faculty. [cited 2007 May 15]. Available from: www.naturaldatabase.com.

- Nemets B, Stahl Z, Belmaker. Addition of omega-3 fatty acid to maintenance medication treatment for recurrent unipolar depressive disorder. Am J Psychiatry. 2003;159:477-9.

- Szegedi A, Kohnen R, Dienel A, Kieser M. Acute treatment of moderate to severe depression with extract WS 5570 (St-John's Wort): randomized controlled double blind non-inferiority trial versus paroxetine. BMJ. 2005; 330:503-8.

- Wilt TJ, Ishani A, Stark G, MacDonald R, Lau Joseph, Mulrow C. Saw Palmetto extracts for treatment of benign prostatic hyperplasia. JAMA. 1998; 280:1604-9.

Units of Measurement

Units of Measurement

Liquid	
1 gallon	3800 mL
1 liquid oz	30 mL
1 teaspoon	5 mL
1 tablespoon	15 mL
1 cup	240 mL
Weight	
1 oz	30 g
1 kg	2.2 lb.
Length	
1 foot	30.48 cm
1 inch	2.54 cm

Laboratory Values: Conversion of American Units into SI Units			
Test	**US Units**	**Conversion Factor**	**SI Units**
Glucose	mg/dL	0.0555	mmol/L
HDL	mg/dL	0.0259	mmol/L
LDL	mg/dL	0.0259	mmol/L
Triglycerides	mg/dL	0.0113	mmol/L

Temperature

- Celsius into Fahrenheit: = (degrees Celsius x 9/5) + 32
- Fahrenheit into Celsius: = (degrees Fahrenheit - 32) x 5/9

References

- Lacy CF, Armstrong LL, Goldman MP, Lance LL, Drug Information Handbook, American Pharmaceutical Association. Lexi-Comp. 8th edition, 2000-2001.
- Institute for Algorithmic Medicine. [Internet]. Medal.org. [cited 2005 March 23]. Available from: http://www.medalreg.com.

Notes

Notes

Notes

_____

_____

_____

_____

_____

_____

_____

_____

_____

_____

_____

_____

_____

_____

_____

Notes

Notes

_____

_____

_____

_____

_____

_____

_____

_____

_____

_____

_____

_____

_____

_____

_____

Notes

Notes

_____

_____

_____

_____

_____

_____

_____

_____

_____

_____

_____

_____

_____

_____

Notes

Notes

_____

_____

_____

_____

_____

_____

_____

_____

_____

_____

_____

_____

_____

_____

_____